Innovation and Invention In Medical Devices

Workshop Summary

Kathi E. Hanna, Frederick J. Manning,
Peter Bouxsein, and Andrew Pope

Editors

Based on a Workshop of the
Roundtable on Research and Development
of Drugs, Biologics, and Medical Devices

Board on Health Sciences Policy

INSTITUTE OF MEDICINE

NATIONAL ACADEMY PRESS
Washington, D.C.

NATIONAL ACADEMY PRESS • 2101 Constitution Avenue, N.W. • Washington, DC 20418

NOTICE: The project that is the subject of this report was approved by the Governing Board of the National Research Council, whose members are drawn from the councils of the National Academy of Sciences, the National Academy of Engineering, and the Institute of Medicine. The members of the committee responsible for the report were chosen for their special competences and with regard for appropriate balance.

Support for this project was provided by the U.S. Department of Health and Human Services and the Greenwall Foundation. The views presented in this report are those of the Institute of Medicine Committee on Assessing the System for Protecting Human Research Subjects and are not necessarily those of the funding agencies.

International Book Standard No. 0-309-08255-2

Additional copies of this report are available for sale from the National Academy Press, 2101 Constitution Avenue, N.W., Box 285, Washington, D.C. 20055. Call (800) 624-6242 or (202) 334-3313 (in the Washington metropolitan area), or visit the NAP's home page at **www.nap.edu**. The full text of this report is available at **www.nap.edu**.

For more information about the Institute of Medicine, visit the IOM home page at **www.iom.edu.**

Copyright 2001 by the National Academy of Sciences. All rights reserved.

Printed in the United States of America.

Knowing is not enough; we must apply.
Willing is not enough; we must do.
—Goethe

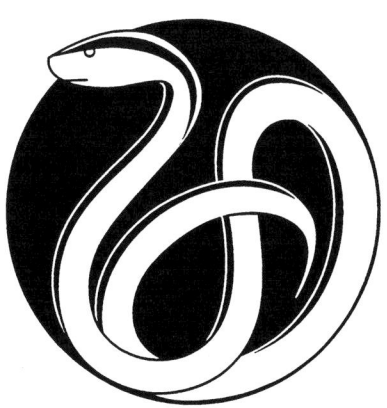

INSTITUTE OF MEDICINE

Shaping the Future for Health

THE NATIONAL ACADEMIES

National Academy of Sciences
National Academy of Engineering
Institute of Medicine
National Research Council

The **National Academy of Sciences** is a private, nonprofit, self-perpetuating society of distinguished scholars engaged in scientific and engineering research dedicated to the furtherance of science and technology and to their use for the general welfare. Upon the authority of the charter granted to it by the Congress in 1863, the Academy has a mandate that requires it to advise the federal government on scientific and technical matters. Dr. Bruce M. Alberts is president of the National Academy of Sciences.

The **National Academy of Engineering** was established in 1964, under the charter of the National Academy of Sciences, as a parallel organization of outstanding engineers. It is autonomous in its administration and in the selection of its members, sharing with the National Academy of Sciences the responsibility for advising the federal government. The National Academy of Engineering also sponsors engineering programs aimed at meeting national needs, encourages education and research, and recognizes the superior achievements of engineers. Dr. Wm. A. Wulf is president of the National Academy of Engineering.

The **Institute of Medicine** was established in 1970 by the National Academy of Sciences to secure the services of eminent members of appropriate professions in the examination of policy matters pertaining to the health of the public. The Institute acts under the responsibility given to the National Academy of Sciences by its congressional charter to be an adviser to the federal government and, upon its own initiative, to identify issues of medical care, research, and education. Dr. Kenneth I. Shine is president of the Institute of Medicine.

The **National Research Council** was organized by the National Academy of Sciences in 1916 to associate the broad community of science and technology with the Academy's purposes of furthering knowledge and advising the federal government. Functioning in accordance with general policies determined by the Academy, the Council has become the principal operating agency of both the National Academy of Sciences and the National Academy of Engineering in providing services to the government, the public, and the scientific and engineering communities. The Council is administered jointly by both Academies and the Institute of Medicine. Dr. Bruce M. Alberts and Dr. Wm. A. Wulf are chairman and vice chairman, respectively, of the National Research Council.

ROUNDTABLE ON RESEARCH AND DEVELOPMENT OF DRUGS, BIOLOGICS, AND MEDICAL DEVICES

RONALD W. ESTABROOK (*Chair*), Virginia Lazenby O'Hara Professor of Biochemistry, University of Texas Southwestern Medical Center, Dallas

ARTHUR L. BEAUDET, Investigator, Howard Hughes Medical Institute, and Professor and Chair, Department of Molecular and Human Genetics, Baylor College of Medicine, Houston, Texas (through February 1999)

LESLIE Z. BENET, Professor and Chair, Department of Biopharmaceutical Sciences, School of Pharmacy, University of California at San Francisco

D. BRUCE BURLINGTON, Director, Center for Devices and Radiological Health, Food and Drug Administration, Rockville, Maryland (through March 1999)

ROBERT CALIFF, Director, Duke Clinical Research Institute, Durham, North Carolina

MICHAEL D. CLAYMAN, Vice President, Global Regulatory Affairs, Lilly Research Laboratories, Indianapolis, Indiana

RITA R. COLWELL, President, Maryland Biotechnology Institute, University of Maryland, College Park (through December 1997)

ADRIAN L. EDWARDS, Private Practice, Internal Medicine/Cardiology, The New York and Presbyterian Hospitals, New York City

DAVID W. FEIGAL, Director, Center for Devices and Radiological Health, Food and Drug Administration, Rockville, Maryland (from June 1999)

STEPHEN GROFT, Director, Office of Rare Diseases Research, National Institutes of Health, Bethesda, Maryland

ANNE B. JACKSON, Sarasota, Florida

ROBERT I. LEVY, Senior Vice President, Science and Technology, American Home Products, Wyeth-Ayerst Research, Madison, New Jersey

MICHAEL R. McGARVEY, Chief Medical Officer, Blue Cross and Blue Shield of New Jersey, Inc., Newark

KSHITIJ MOJAN, Corporate Vice President for Research and Technical Services, Baxter Health Care Corporation, Roundlake, Illinois

STUART L. NIGHTINGALE, Associate Commissioner, Health Affairs, Food and Drug Administration, Rockville, Maryland

PAUL GRANT ROGERS, Partner, Hogan & Hartson, Washington, D.C.

DANIEL SECKINGER, Group Vice President, Professional Standards, American Medical Association, Chicago, Illinois (through December 1997)

WHAIJEN SOO, Vice President, Clinical Sciences, Roche Pharmaceuticals, Hoffmann-La Roche, Inc., Nutley, New Jersey

REED TUCKSON, Group Vice President, Professional Standards, American Medical Association, Chicago, Illinois (from October 1998)

JANET WOODCOCK, Director, Center for Drug Evaluation and Research, Food and Drug Administration, Rockville, Maryland

SUMNER YAFFE, Director, Center for Research for Mothers and Children, National Institute of Child Health and Human Development, National Institutes of Health, Bethesda, Maryland

KATHRYN ZOON, Director, Center for Biologics Evaluation and Research, Food and Drug Administration, Rockville, Maryland

Liaisons to the Roundtable

C. THOMAS CASKEY, Senior Vice President for Research, Merck & Co., Inc., West Point, Pennsylvania

JAMES S. BENSON, Executive Vice President, Technology and Regulatory Affairs, Health Industry Manufacturers Association, Washington, D.C.

BRIAN J. MALKIN, Associate Director for Patents and Hearings, Office of Health Affairs, Food and Drug Administration, Rockville, Maryland

BERT SPILKER, Senior Vice President, Scientific and Regulatory Affairs, Pharmaceutical Research and Manufacturers of America, Washington, D.C.

Study Staff

JONATHAN R. DAVIS, Senior Program Officer
VIVIAN P. NOLAN, Research Associate
CHRISTINA THACKER, Research Assistant (to July 1998)
NICOLE AMADO, Project Assistant

Division Staff

ANDREW M. POPE, Division Director
LINDA DEPUGH, Administrative Assistant
JAMAINE TINKER, Financial Associate (to October 1998)
CARLOS GABRIEL, Financial Associate (from February 1999)

REVIEWERS

This report has been reviewed in draft form by individuals chosen for their diverse perspectives and technical expertise, in accordance with procedures approved by the NRC's Report Review Committee. The purpose of this independent review is to provide candid and critical comments that will assist the institution in making its published report as sound as possible and to ensure that the report meets institutional standards for objectivity, evidence, and responsiveness to the study charge. The review comments and draft manuscript remain confidential to protect the integrity of the deliberative process. We wish to thank the following individuals for their review of this report:

Clifford Goodman, The Lewin Group
Robert Mann, Massachusetts Institute of Technology
Richard A. Merrill, University of Virginia School of Law
Daniel Wooten, Institute of Medicine

Although the reviewers listed above have provided many constructive comments and suggestions, they were not asked to endorse the conclusions or recommendations nor did they see the final draft of the report before its release. The review of this report was overseen by **Melvin Worth**, Institute of Medicine. Appointed by the Institute of Medicine, he was responsible for making certain that an independent examination of this report was carried out in accordance with institutional procedures and that all review comments were carefully considered. Responsibility for the final content of this report rests entirely with the authoring committee and the institution.

Foreword

Kenneth I. Shine, M.D.
President, Institute of Medicine

As a cardiologist I have had experience with many medical devices. The experience that had the most profound effect on me was as a medical student caring for a young man with what was called the Hufnagle valve, a "birdcage" valve that was placed in the descending aorta in patients who had aortic insufficiency. It was placed in the descending aorta because at the time Hufnagle developed it we did not have the techniques to allow placing the valve directly into aortic position. Thus, it was done through a thoracotomy. It did not affect the regurgitation in the upper portion of the body, only in the lower portion.

What was remarkable about this device was that it made noise. It was located close to the trachea, and if a patient opened his mouth, people across the room could hear the clicking. As long as the patient was in sinus rhythm, they could tolerate the noise, but over time some of these patients developed atrial fibrillation, which produced a random clicking that was highly disturbing to them. The patient I took care of committed suicide because he could no longer tolerate the sound.

Much progress has been made with prosthetic valves since that time. The Hufnagle valve was an extraordinary contribution at the time that it was first implanted, but it had unexpected limitations. Development of medical devices depends on innovation that moves the field safely forward in a way that continually improves over time.

The Roundtable on Research and Development of Drugs, Biologics, and Medical Devices has provided a useful forum for the exchange of ideas and concerns among representatives of industry, government, and academia. This communication has enhanced the performance of all three sectors. Institute of Medicine roundtables are relatively unique in that they provide an opportunity for industry, government, and academia to come together over time to confront important issues. The Roundtable has had two previous workshops, one exploring issues regarding the quality and validity of data generated by clinical trials, and the other examining how to improve the quality and quantity of therapeutics developed and dispensed to infants and children. In April 2000, the IOM launched the National Clinical Research Roundtable to bring together individuals concerned about the future of clinical research.

This particular workshop focuses on medical devices at an exciting and challenging time, when the field is diverse, covering a range of implants, imaging equipment, surgical instruments, prosthetics, and orthotics. One of the challenges to the field derives from the rapidly expanding science base. This expansion is bound to continue or even accelerate given the kind of projected increases in the budgets of the National Institutes of Health and the National Science Foundation. The challenge is to make sure that the science base is reflected in the development of new devices and that we learn new ways to blend engineering and medicine.

The flip side of that challenge is to make sure that newly developed devices are responsive to the most pressing needs of patients. There is a continuing debate over how much medical device innovation really is pioneering and how much is embellishing existing devices and making them more costly. I remind you of the fundamental changes taking place in the pharmaceutical industry, in which the more mature companies have determined that it is no longer profitable for them to develop "me-too" drugs. The types of drugs that will make substantial profits are those that come first to market. This change in approach is going to have implications for the device industry as well.

A second major challenge is to ensure that beneficial innovations are made available to patients in need. It is extremely difficult to predict how the device field will develop over the next several years, let alone how insurance companies, managed care companies, and government programs are going to deal with these changes. Who is going to pay for what and in what manner? One thing I am fairly certain about is that patients, physicians, and payers are going to be looking for value. They are weary of the continued escalation in health care costs and the contributions to these costs made by medical devices. We cannot ignore the fact that the quality of the innovation must be measured not only by what it can do but also by its incremental costs and benefits. We must conduct rigorous evidence-based evaluations of the safety, efficacy, and relative effectiveness of health care technologies to ensure that our limited health care dollars are spent as effectively as possible in promoting overall health.

In the field of devices, we need a better nosology, that is, the classification of devices, and we need to determine how each class of device should be evaluated for approval purposes and long-term follow-up. My concern here is that for most individuals and groups working on devices, evaluation tends to be very much tailored to the particular device, which makes it extraordinarily difficult to figure out what types of data are necessary to be compelling. We need to do a better job with classification so that investigators and regulators have a clearer notion of the expectations for the approval and follow-up processes. This workshop explores the challenges, opportunities, and obstacles facing the field of medical devices.

Preface

The Institute of Medicine Roundtable on Research and Development of Drugs, Biologics, and Medical Devices has evolved from the Forum on Drug Development, established in 1986. The importance of maintaining a neutral setting for discussions regarding long-term and politically sensitive issues was determined by sponsor representatives and the Institute of Medicine to justify the need for revising and enhancing past efforts. The new Roundtable is intended to be a convening mechanism for dialogue and exchange of information among individuals, including government officials, who represent all sides of public policy issues related to the development of drugs, biologics, and medical devices.

Goals of the Roundtable include providing an environment for the exchange of information and the identification of high priority issues in the areas of product discovery and development. In order to achieve these goals, the Roundtable convenes twice annually in Washington, D.C., and holds at least one workshop each year.

Members of the Roundtable bring expertise from clinical medicine, pharmacology, health policy, industrial management, and product development as they pertain to research and development of drugs, biologics, and medical devices. Each member's participation adds a unique perspective to discussion topics. Members are responsible for identifying areas of Roundtable focus and issues that can be further elucidated in subsequent workshops. These workshops provide the opportunity to assemble a broader group of experts in the area of interest.

The Roundtable identifies problems that are current and likely to be ongoing, or expected to arise within the next few years, and develops approaches to exploit opportunities or solve problems. Previous workshops have focused on assuring data quality and review in the conduct and review of clinical trials and issues in pediatric drug development. The first two were *Assuring Data Quality and Validity in Clinical Trials for Regulatory Decision Making* and *Rational Therapeutics for Infants and Children*. This, the third workshop, focuses on innovation and invention in medical devices. To allow full and candid participation, through this workshop, the Roundtable's goal was not to make recommendations or endorse specific courses of action, but to identify approaches that can or might be used to promote innovation in the medical devices area.

The early stage of the innovation process involves matching technologies to needs, and sometimes the matching of technology to needs gets done through technology push. Sometimes it is achieved through demand pull. The different disciplines represented at this workshop are those that intersect at various points in the innovation process, and the challenge is the extent to which that intersection can be managed. Can it be productive without taking away the essential tensions required, yet allow synergistic and constructive progress?

Traditionally the intersections of medicine, engineering, materials science, and electronics have been the focus of device development. That development is now growing. Molecular biology and immunology have entered the *in vitro* diagnostics area, as well as implants and prosthetics. These new intersections cause researchers to stop and ask whether these products are devices, drugs, or biologics? Thus, these advances challenge traditional paradigms.

Researchers are also challenged by the need to evaluate the contributions that devices make to improved health and to costs. With drugs, there is a massive upfront cost but the incremental cost of the next pill is small. The relationship to health outcome is often more obvious for drugs than in the case of devices. The complications with the delivery and use of devices are very different. The unit cost of devices can be very low or extremely high. Because of the wide range of devices and their costs, developing a device economic model is not simple, although it is a worthy goal. At the end of all these intersections is one common goal; to find solutions and answers to mitigate the adverse human condition.

Ronald W. Estabrook, Ph.D.	Kshitij Mohan, Ph.D.
Roundtable Chair	Workshop Chair

Acronyms and Abbreviations

AdvaMed	Advanced Medical Technology Association (formerly Health Industry Manufacturers Association [HIMA])
APL	Advanced Physics Lab
ATD	Advanced Technology Development
BECON	Bioengineering Consortium
CBER	Center for Biologics Evaluation and Research
CDC	Centers for Disease Control and Prevention
CDER	Center for Drug Evaluation and Research
CDRH	Center for Devices and Radiologic Health
CIEBM	Committee on the Interplay of Engineering with Biology and Medicine
CIMIT	Center for Innovative Minimally Invasive Therapy
CMS	Centers for Medicare and Medicaid Services (formerly Health Care Financing Administration [HCFA])
CPT	Current Procedural Technology
CTO	Commercial Technology Office
DHHS	Department of Health and Human Services
DPI	Dry Powder Inhaler

EU	European Union
FDA	Food and Drug Administration
GMP	Good Manufacturing Practice
HCFA	Health Care Financing Administration (now Centers for Medicare and Medicaid Services [CMS])
HIMA	Health Industry Manufacturers Association (now Advanced Medical Technology Association [AdvaMed])
ICG	Impedance Cardiography
ICH	International Conference on Harmonisation of Technical Requirements for Registration of Pharmaceuticals for Human Use
IDE	Investigational Device Exemption
IND	Investigational New Drug
IOM	Institute of Medicine
IRB	Institutional Review Board
ISS	International Space Station
LAVD	Left Ventricle Assist Device
MDI	Metered Dose Inhaler
MDN	Medical Device Network
MDR	Medical Device Report
MEMS	Micro-Electromechanical Systems
MIC	Minnesota Impedance Cardiograph
MIT	Massachusetts Institute of Technology
MWGC	MultiWire Gamma Camera
NAE	National Academy of Engineering
NDA	New Drug Applications
NIH	National Institutes of Health
NIST	National Institute of Standards and Technology
NSF	National Science Foundation
OCT	Optical Coherence Tomography
OPS	Orthogonal Polarization Spectral
PCR	Polymerase Chain Reaction
PCT	Patent Cooperation Treaty
PICAB	Percutaneous in Situ Coronary Artery Bypass Grafting

PMA	Premarketing Approval
PQRI	Product Quality Research Institute
PTH	Parathyroid Hormone
SBIR	Small Business Innovative Research
SNP	Single Nucleotide Polymorphism
Ta-178	Tantalum-178
TIP	Telemedicine Instrumentation Pack
TMR	Transmyocardial Revascularization

Contents

1 **INTRODUCTORY OVERVIEW** 1
Overview, 1
Challenges to Innovation, 2
Regulatory Issues, 3
Payment Issues, 4
Value and Consequences for Innovation, 7
Conclusions, 7

2 **KEYNOTE SESSION** 9
Historical Perspective on IOM's Role in Providing a Forum for
    Discussion, 9
A Regulatory Perspective, 13
An Industry Perspective: Challenges in the Development and
    Regulation of Drug-Device Combination Products, 16
An Evaluator's Perspective, 20
Innovation and Invention in Medical Devices: Implantable
    Defibrillators, 21
General Discussion of the Keynote Session, 25

3 **THE NATURE OF MEDICAL INNOVATION** 31
The Innovative Process for Medical Devices: A NASA
    Perspective, 31
Endovascular Devices, 36
Gene Arrays, 39

     Inhaled Insulin, 40
     Imaging the Microvasculature, 41
     General Discussion of the Nature of Medical Innovation, 43

4 SOURCES AND SUPPORT OF MEDICAL DEVICES INNOVATION 47
     An Overview of Public and Private Factors Affecting Medical Device Innovation, 47
     The Federal Research Role, 49
     The Federal Regulatory Role, 50
     The Academic Role in Innovation, 51
     The Academic Health Center Environment, 52
     The Role of Small Medical Companies, 54
     The Role of Large Medical Companies, 54
     The Role of Public and Private Capital, 56
     General Discussion of Sources and Support of Medical Device Innovation, 57

5 THE CHALLENGES AHEAD 61
     Unmet Clinical Needs: Cardiovascular Disease, 61
     Unmet Clinical Needs: Clinical Trials, 63
     Barriers and Issues in Device Innovation: Reimbursement, 64
     General Discussion of the Challenges Ahead, 65

6 SUMMARY AND CONCLUSIONS 69

APPENDIXES
A Workshop Agenda, 71
B Speakers' Biographical Sketches, 77
C Registered Participants, 89

1

Introductory Overview

The objective of the workshop that is the subject of this summary report was to present the challenges and opportunities for medical devices as perceived by the key stakeholders in the field. The agenda, and hence the summaries of the presentations that were made in the workshop and which are presented in this summary report, was organized to first examine the nature of innovation in the field and the social and economic infrastructure that supports such innovation. The next objective was to identify and discuss the greatest unmet clinical needs, with a futuristic view of technologies that might meet those needs. And finally, consideration was given to the barriers to the application of new technologies to meet clinical needs.

OVERVIEW
Harry M. Jansen Kraemer, Jr.
Chairman and Chief Executive Officer
Baxter International, Inc.

Medical devices have extended the ability of physicians to diagnose and treat diseases, making great contributions to health and quality of life. Beyond the considerable attention that such big-ticket technologies as computer-assisted tomography and magnetic resonance imaging have received, there is no doubt that these technologies have changed the mainstream practice of medicine. However, diagnostic technology is not limited to capital equipment imagers. It also includes analytical techniques using high-resolution chromatography, polymerase chain reaction (PCR), and monoclonal antibodies, providing physicians with new, accurate, and rapid information.

On the therapeutic side, devices save lives and improve quality of life. Dialysis therapy extends lives for end-stage renal disease patients, orthopedic implants enable patients to walk again, and minimally invasive technologies allow surgeries that are safer, with less pain and trauma, requiring significantly shorter hospital stays.

The United States is clearly the leader in medical device innovation. In 1998, the United States medical device and diagnostics industry was responsible for nearly $70 billion in production, which is almost 50% of the total world consumption of medical technology. The United States exports significantly more devices than it imports, netting a trade surplus of almost $10 billion. Further, United States medical device patents outnumber foreign patents by more than three to one.

What makes the United States system so special? Kraemer believes that a fundamental part of the success of the United States is that it is a society that promotes and rewards innovation. The United States has a strong science base and an entrepreneurial culture of sophisticated and efficient financial markets, intellectual property protection, and a health care system that for the most part has been willing to pay for technological advances.

CHALLENGES TO INNOVATION

Despite being the best system in the world, however, the United States faces major challenges that can undermine the viability of innovation and access to better health care. One striking characteristic is that medical device innovation often requires the contributions of a diverse array of scientific and engineering expertise. Something as seemingly basic as the materials used in medical products, for example, have made lasting contributions to health care in ways people often take for granted. For example, the first plastic blood collection container enhanced the safety and quality of stored blood and made possible the separation of individual blood components. Thus, modern blood component transfusion therapy was made possible by plastics. Miniaturized circuitry for pacemakers, mathematical algorithms used in MRI, and greater understanding of fluid mechanics for heart valves were all developed outside the conventional areas of medical research.

Obviously researchers cannot script innovation. At times it occurs in a great stroke of luck or insight. At other times it is a gradual process with new devices piggy-backing off earlier ones. Innovation extends well beyond laboratories, including the many instances of clinicians finding new indications for already-launched technology, as well as breakthroughs that have occurred at the intersection of multiple scientific and technical streams of progress.

An example of an early innovation that continues to find new applications in medicine is the laser. Invented in 1958, the laser was first applied in health care as a non-contact scalpel. New applications of lasers include reshaping corneas, photodynamic therapy for cancer, and transmyocardial revascularization (TMR) for severe angina. TMR for severe angina exemplifies the tremendous uncertainty at the leading edge of innovation. Despite its apparent early success, researchers are still not sure if it really works and, if it does, how. It also highlights an important aspect of innovation: the timing and methodological rigor of clinical trials to test innovations and the relation of these to regulation and payment for new technology.

Innovation requires time, insight, and sometimes luck. It also requires significant financial resources. What do researchers currently do to create an environment that is conducive to innovation?

First, the United States has a strong commitment to basic science, which forms the basis for future innovations. The United States funds more basic research than the next six countries combined. The National Institutes of Health (NIH) and the National Science Foundation (NSF) granted extramural funds of more than $13 billion in 1998 alone to support the sciences. Advances in basic sciences, such as understanding of genetics, biology, physics, and chemistry, enable the rapid pace of innovation.

This interaction between scientist, engineer, and clinician can be further promoted to speed the process of innovation. Although it is the single most prolific and important biomedical research entity in the world, NIH is organized primarily into disease- and organ-specific institutes in a way that is less than optimally supportive of technological disciplines that cut across institute priorities. While some institutes do invest in engineering tools and techniques, these are specific to institute priorities and do not sufficiently support the underlying science and engineering that spawn future advances in health care technology.

Support for biomedical engineering in the private sector is considerably greater than support by the government, and nearly all of the private sector investment is devoted to applied research. Shoring up the federal investment, particularly for basic research, would strengthen our national capacity for technological innovation.

Researchers increasingly understand that innovation is more than producing the latest widget. The downstream hurdles of regulation and payment affect not only whether a device gets on the market and becomes accessible to patients, but they also send feedback to the process of innovation itself. If the regulatory process is perceived as being slow and expensive for innovative devices, then incentives shift to produce more "me-too," or derivative, devices that may have a less risky road to market.

REGULATORY ISSUES

For reasons both fair and unfair, the Food and Drug Administration (FDA) has been cited over the years as a major barrier to innovation. Kraemer is among the first to state that FDA, and specifically the Center for Devices and Radiological Health, have taken many important measures to streamline regulatory processes, making them more transparent and predictable. This is not to say that interactions with FDA cannot be significantly improved. In fact, it may be somewhat ironic that the pendulum may have swung too far toward transparency, with the potential for confidential information to be released by the agency over the objections of industry. Still, rather than view FDA as an adversary, Kraemer would like to point out that researchers all share the goal of improving patients' lives at the same time that they minimize the risks.

The most important issue, the one that researchers have all grappled with is that of over-regulation versus adequate regulation. The agency has acknowledged that devices are different than drugs. In general, devices have faster cycle times and tend to be characterized by incremental improvements, leading to longer-run significant advances. As such, earlier devices can provide considerable bases of information on the safety and efficacy of the next generation. It is difficult to have placebo controls in clinical trials of most devices or to double-blind physicians and patients as to who is getting which technology. Moreover, given the sizes of the target populations for many devices, it can be impractical to conduct randomized clinical trials with devices as they are done for drugs. Thus, clinical trial requirements and designs must reflect the technology at hand. And, whether for drugs or devices, there are always practical and ethical challenges of informed consent.

Clearly, devices need to be regulated differently than drugs, and FDA is increasingly aware of this. Even so, researchers have far to go in pursuit of the least burdensome provision of the FDA Modernization Act of 1997. There remain inefficiencies due to unnecessary regulatory impediments.

A fascinating and important issue arises out of the rapid evolution of technology itself, that is, the fit between new forms of technology and the FDA jurisdiction over technology. For regulatory purposes, how should xenotransplants—in which animal organs are genetically engineered to express human surface proteins, thereby suppressing rejection—be classified? Are they devices or are they biologics? Should they be regulated by the Center for Devices and Radiological Health or the Center for Biologics Evaluation and Research?

Under what model of regulation should these hybrids fall, and how prepared is the agency for handling this technology? This jurisdictional issue involves not only FDA but also the Centers for Disease Control and Prevention (CDC) and institutional review boards. In any case, a technology company that is weighing whether to push forward in innovative areas must consider the time and risk involved as well as the hurdles and other procedural matters.

PAYMENT ISSUES

Payment issues are of increasing concern to the health care industry. Everybody talks about the rising costs of health care and the need to find ways of managing costs more effectively. In fact, some continue to point to technology as a major culprit in increasing costs. To the extent that technology continues to improve health and quality of life for more people, it is not clear to Kraemer that people are spending too much on health care. Nevertheless, the emphasis on cost and the role of technology in costs have placed part of the onus on the industry.

It is part of corporate consciousness that innovation is not just creating a better widget. It includes creating more cost-effective alternatives to current therapies. Of course, it is not quite that simple. There is increasing emphasis on cost-effectiveness as a yardstick for payment. While payers here in the United States and in other industrialized nations say that they are interested in cost-effectiveness, too often it appears that their interest is just plain cost cutting.

Cost is in the equation, but where are the benefits to health in that equation? In this environment, providers are getting pressured to use cost-saving technology as opposed to cost-effective technology. Manufacturers are under pressure to consolidate, to make technologies into commodities, and to compete on the basis of price alone. A major factor contributing to United States leadership is the willingness to pay for proven innovation. Price fixing and rationing, which are used in other nations, fail to account for the effectiveness side of the equation.

What are the incentives for innovators to start new companies and for manufacturers to invest in new technologies? What is the trade-off of risk for expected return on investment? It may be one thing for producing those commodity widgets and their costs. It is another for taking on the risk often required to create technologies that may have higher price tags but may yield significant leaps in health outcomes.

Part of what makes this business so complicated as well as personally gratifying is the obligation to help people who are making decisions about their parents, spouses, or children. People's perspectives change significantly depending on whether they are dealing with abstract statistical populations or with their family, when cost does not matter and arguments that a technology is not cost-saving or cost-effective often fall on deaf ears. This affects the policy debate and the likelihood of success of policy initiatives regarding health care technology. It is a complicated issue that must be addressed.

There are, however, payment issues that can be addressed in the short term. Kraemer refers to the daunting task of navigating the maze of public- and private-sector payers within health care. Although FDA can be a tough customer, at least there is only one FDA. There are many parties that affect payment—the multiple Medicare carriers, state Medicaid programs, the Blues, Aetna, United Healthcare, Kaiser, Cigna—all with varying requirements and different approvals for payment. Kraemer in no way advocates the adoption of a single-payer system, but from the perspective of technology companies, the prospect of getting over the FDA hurdle just to face a multitude of payers is not a pretty sight. It does figure significantly into the risk equation.

One payer that continues to be highly influential is Medicare. Medicare is not necessarily the first to make a payment decision, but when it does decide to cover a new technology, it puts a lot of pressure on all the other payers. When Medicare does not cover a new technology it makes it easier for other payers not to make a positive coverage decision. The Medicare coverage process is a challenge to many companies. After FDA approval, the biggest concern for a manufacturer of an innovative device is denial of coverage. New devices that are improvements on earlier versions do not necessarily have this problem. As long as they are not great departures from their predecessors, the next stent or the next pacemaker has a much clearer road for achieving reimbursement.

Barriers to coverage can affect innovation in at least two ways. First, startups and manufacturers concerned about the risk of coverage denial may prefer to invest in safer next-generation technologies instead of breakthrough technologies. Second, innovation does not stop when a device hits the market. Devices can be refined over time, and applied to different indications to find unexpected uses. An early coverage denial not only holds back a technology for its original use and refinement, but it delays or eliminates opportunities for identifying other beneficial indications.

The situation has brightened for payment during clinical trials. Prior to 1995, it was Medicare's policy to deny payment for virtually all non-FDA-approved devices and off-label uses, even those with predicates with proven safety and efficacy. This posed a significant disincentive for innovation by raising costs for manufacturers and making providers reluctant to participate in clinical trials. In 1995, the Health Care Financing Administration (HCFA)[1] and FDA agreed to an approach for classifying new devices into those that are truly novel and those that are basically next-generation versions, and making the latter categories eligible for Medicare reimbursement. This 1995 interagency agreement is an example of a strong collaborative step in the right direction for improving technology payment as well as access.

Payment problems remain, however, including the process of coding and securing adequate payment for use of medical devices. A new device needs a new Current Procedural Technology (CPT) code to make sure that doctors can be reimbursed. Even with a proper code, the Medicare payment level for that code may not be sufficient to cover the cost of the procedure and the technology it embodies, thereby constituting a significant disincentive for doctors to use the device. This entire coverage and coding process can take years from the time a product is launched (unless the new device already has a code in place), but the payment level is so low as to be a significant disincentive for doctors to use it. These payment hurdles are significant for large technology companies, but they are especially daunting to smaller companies that do not have the dedicated staff, experience, and other resources to handle these issues effectively.

What can be done in the short term to address these issues? HCFA recently revamped its national Medicare coverage process and is still working out some problems. However, HCFA also needs to reform its processes and requirements regarding coding and payment levels to make these much more timely, transparent, and fair. FDA and HCFA can cooperate to reduce duplication of effort significantly and streamline processes.

---

[1] Now Center for Medicare and Medicaid Services (CMS).

VALUE AND CONSEQUENCES FOR INNOVATION

The need to demonstrate clinical and economic value is a central issue in regulation and payment, and it is clear that the trend is toward requiring more evidence rather than less for innovative devices. However, building evidence of value can be costly and time-consuming, and at some point reaches diminishing returns with respect to the availability and benefits of the technology.

In an ideal world, a decision maker has definitive proof that the device will improve health outcomes, be less costly, or improve outcomes at an acceptable cost, but that certainty comes with lost or delayed opportunities to improve people's health and the quality of life. These trade-offs look very different depending on who a person is. If a person is a government agency charged with protecting against potential health hazards of something new, or charged with minding the public purse, it may make sense to err on the side of delay, but from the perspective of some patients and their doctors, that same delay can be a life and death proposition.

Even when researchers have enough evidence to understand the safety, efficacy, and cost of a device, the interpretation of value can vary depending on perspective, including those of patients, hospitals, managed care organizations, technology assessment agencies, the government, and society at large. For many of these perspectives, it is hard to argue against a device that works, reduces complications, saves lives, and costs less than the alternatives, but most of the time it is not quite that easy.

Left ventricular assist devices (LVADs) are a great example. Each year there are at least 60,000 patients with severe heart failure unresponsive to medical therapy who need a heart transplant, but who are unable to get one, due to either their age or other complications. Many do not get transplants simply because there are so few donor hearts available. Only about 2,500 patients, or less than 5%, get heart transplants each year. LVADs were developed as a bridge to cardiac transplantation for patients with severe heart failure. The need for LVADs is clear. They are proven, and they were approved recently by FDA. These devices clearly are not cheap. They can range from $45,000 to $65,000 per unit and, as is the case with so many medical devices, people tend to focus on the price tag. End-stage heart disease is not cheap, but its price tag is harder to discern and, unfortunately, end-stage means exactly that, end-stage. The potential of LVADs as bridges to transplant was limited by the number of available hearts. Now, given the continued shortage of heart donors, LVADs are in clinical trials as alternatives rather than bridges to cardiac replacement. This changes the size of the potential patient target population and changes the potential costs for payers. It will be interesting to see how this all plays out.

CONCLUSIONS

Society places a high premium on innovation. Patients expect and demand that researchers will continue to develop cures for an aging population. The public wants the latest breakthroughs—not in years or in months, but today. Increasingly, researchers want and expect patients to be more interested, more informed, and more active about making health care choices, but the counterpoint to patient activism is patience with the time it takes to achieve that new breakthrough.

Can the current system continue to support these expectations? The promise of new developments in biotechnology, genetics, tissue engineering and, of course, computers and the Internet are transforming the industry, but researchers must continue to survey the innovation landscape and manage those hurdles, potholes, and inclement weather.

Chief among these issues is society's definition of value and the evidence researchers will accept to prove that value. Researchers recognize that the process and products of innovation will continue to be tested. The bar is set high. Researchers need ongoing dialogue from all perspectives to define and redefine as necessary what they must achieve in clinical benefits and how they are willing to pay for these benefits. Solutions may not be easy and no one has all the answers, but it is at gatherings like this that researchers can put the issues on the table, provide practical and constructive review, and promote action to achieve their shared purpose of improving the health and quality of life for every American.

2

Keynote Session

This chapter contains summaries of the individual presentations from the keynote session of the Workshop. The objective was to hear from key stakeholders from research, clinical practice, regulatory agencies, and industry in order to provide their perspectives on innovation and invention in the medical device industry.

HISTORICAL PERSPECTIVE ON IOM'S ROLE IN PROVIDING A FORUM FOR DISCUSSION

Robert W. Mann, Sc.D.
Whitaker Professor Emeritus of Biomedical Engineering
Massachusetts Institute of Technology

The inaugural national effort addressing the issues this Workshop is considering was the Committee on the Interplay of Engineering with Biology and Medicine (CIEBM),[1] established in 1967 by the National Academy of Engineering (NAE) "to delineate the means by which the national engineering capability can be effectively applied to biology, medicine, and health services." Collaboration between practitioners of medicine and engineering in the Institute of Medicine (IOM) was insured at its inception in 1970 by charter provisions[2] de-

---

[1] "An Assessment of Industrial Activity in the Field of Biomedical Engineering," Appendix A, National Academy of Engineering, Washington, D.C., 1971.

[2] Charter section "II Membership 1. The membership of the Institute shall consist of persons selected from the fields of health and medicine ... and from such other fields related to health and medicine as the ... medical and biological sciences ... and engineering." The physical sciences are not specifically mentioned.

fining the membership. In the early 1970s, the IOM Committee on Science Policy for Medicine and Health established as a priority interdisciplinary research collaboration between the life sciences and medicine and the physical sciences and engineering, including the innovation of medical devices. In the early 1980s, further activities facilitated interdisciplinary interactions between the physical sciences and medicine, including the formation of a Working Group on Interdisciplinary Collaboration, also supported by the Whitaker Foundation, and a Committee on Promoting Research Collaboration. Topics addressed by these groups included federal policy, the academic-industrial interface, the role of private foundations, and the role of university and teaching hospital structures in facilitating interdisciplinary research. *Interdisciplinary Research: Promoting Collaboration Between the Life Sciences and Medicine and the Physical Sciences and Engineering* was published in 1990, stating that, "The committee recognized two different motivations for collaborative research: (1) the desire to increase understanding of natural phenomena, and (2) the need to provide practical benefits."

To address directly "practical benefits" in terms of new medical devices and explore important issues and interrelationships of engineering, medicine, invention, and public policy, the NAE and IOM, in their first major collaborative effort, jointly convened the symposium, *New Medical Devices: Factors Influencing Invention, Development, and Use,* in March 1987. The symposium brought physicians, engineers, and scientists together with industry executives, lawyers, ethicists, economists, and government officials to explore key factors that would influence development and use of innovative medical devices during the next decade. Symposium participants identified current trends in federal and private support of technological innovation, medical device regulation, product liability, and health care reimbursement. In addition, participants addressed important general issues, such as how to sustain technological innovation and health care quality in a rapidly changing health care environment, and how to encourage and support inventors.

After the highly successful symposium, in 1988 the National Academy Press published *New Medical Devices: Invention, Development and Use*, which addressed the three major themes: (1) innovation and use of new medical devices; (2) current trends in federal and private support of technological innovation, medical device regulation, product liability, and health care reimbursement; and (3) several perspectives on how these trends interact to influence the availability and appropriate use of new medical devices.

At the 1988 symposium, five inventors reported that basic science advances were of little direct relevance in their innovation of Technion's Auto Analyzer, plasmapheresis, the pneumatic extradural intracranial pressure monitor, the electronic retinoscope, the first successful implantable cardiac pacemaker, and wheelchairs for the third world. Edward B. Roberts of the Massachusetts Institute of Technology (MIT) Sloan School, said "innovation in medical devices is usually based on engineering problem-solving by individuals or small firms, is often incremental rather than radical, seldom depends on the results of long-term research in the basic sciences, and generally does not reflect the recent generation of fundamental new knowledge." Medical device innovation was reported to be quite different from that of the pharmaceutical industry, where basic research is carried out in large organizations, generating fundamental knowledge in order to create radical drug innovations.

Has the intervening decade changed the earlier assessment, specifically with respect to traditional medical devices, those employing mechano-electrical-electronic-magnetic technologies? To get a sense of what the answer might be, Dr. Mann polled colleagues involved in devising new medical devices and consistently was told that once demand is recognized or anticipated and concept conceived, the process is intrinsically engineering problem solving, evaluation, improvement, and practical and economic manufacture, not to mention finding funding and addressing marketing issues. Clinical trials are expensive and take a long time. Certainly this process is true for medical devices widely deployed, for example, single-use endoscopic instruments, artificial hip and knee joints, stents, and intraocular lenses. The same process applies to even less common instruments, such as the left-ventricular assist device,[3] and cochlear implants, and those under development, such as visual prostheses.[4]

Given the existing cornucopia of physics- and chemistry-based engineering science knowledge, and so many powerful processes and techniques—such as computer-aided design/computer-aided manufacturing, robotics, VLSI chips, and microfab—there is no need for designers of traditional devices to mount or seek basic research.

Dr. Mann offered two contemporary examples of what he calls traditional medical devices. The first is an epiretinal implant to stimulate the ganglion cells of the eye to reverse the progress of blindness in macular degeneration.[5] Major problems cited by the innovators were the insertion into, and mechanical compatibility of the stimulating implant with the retina, which they describe as "like a sheet of wet Kleenex." These are both basically design problems, and concern long-term biocompatibility. Dr. Mann's second example involves a cardiac surgeon seated at a computer 3-D display of the patient's heart, moving a manipulandum as he would during open-heart surgery to repair a defective heart valve. This complex employs systems integration and ergonomic design of stereoscopic imaging with optical magnification and tiny robots, combined with an endoscope inserted through centimeter-sized slits in the patient's chest. The device, manipulated by the surgeon and aided by multi-sensory feedback, is minimally invasive.[6]

---

[3] "The LVAD: A Case Study," Victor L. Poirier, *The Bridge,* Volume 27, Number 4, Winter 1997, pp. 14–20, NAE.

[4] "Retinal Prostheses," Joseph. F. Rizzo III and John Wyatt, Chapter 25, *Age-Related Macular Degeneration,* Mosby, St. Louis.

[5] "Prospects for a Visual Prostheses," Joseph. F. Rizzo III and John Wyatt, *The Neuroscientist,* Volume 3, Number 4, 1997, pp. 251–262.

[6] "The Heart of Microsurgery," J. Kenneth Salisbury, *Mechanical Engineering,* December 1998, pp. 46–51.

In the 1988 report, Dr. Mann's foreword stated, "In my opinion, the research areas grievously underserved are interdisciplinary questions undergirding future medical devices. We have run the string of devices nostalgically described by our inventors. Future medical technology will increasingly require more fundamental understanding at the organ, cell, and subcellular levels, and it will be based on collaborative biological and physical science research." At that time, a number of new areas were emerging, including biomaterials, biosensors, artificial organs, and functional neurostimulation. To today's list can be added tissue engineering,[7] developing biological substitutes for natural tissues—skin or cartilage for example—and ultimately organ transplants, interdigitation of molecular biology and engineering systems analysis through computational modeling of biological systems at the molecular level to understand metabolism, adhesion, mechanical contraction proliferation, differentiation, and molecule-to-cell and cell-to-cell signaling.[8] The more holistic tissue engineering and more reductionist modeling will in time converge, leading to a more fundamentally based realization of medical devices, to have a profound positive capability to promote, regain, and extend human health.

The intervening decade has seen a dramatic increase in university programs, departments, and curricula in bioengineering,[9] driven partly by the emergence of biology as a subject common to undergraduate education and partly by the generous and dedicated funding contributed to bioengineering and biomedical engineering programs by the Whitaker Foundation.[10] The more than 70 biomedical engineering departments and programs in the United States have benefited greatly from the $540 million in grants from Whitaker in the past two decades, but how this large enterprise will be sustained when Whitaker spends itself out in 2006 as planned remains to be seen. Dr. Mann added that federal support for the area has always been modest and peer review committees have not been broadly cognizant of the merits of generous support of the field. The American Institute of Medical and Biological Engineering, composed of academic, governmental, and industrial practitioners with academic, society, and industrial councils, was inaugurated in 1992 to enhance the visibility of the field and lobby for more federal funding, especially from NIH.[11] In April 2001, the National Institute of Biomedical Imaging and Bioengineering was established at NIH.

---

[7] "Tissue Engineering: Confronting the Transplantation Crisis," Robert M. Nerem, Proceedings of the Institute of Mechanical Engineering [H]. 2000;214(1):95–9.

[8] "Engineering Cell Function," by Douglas A. Lauffenburger, *The Bridge,* Volume 27, Number 4, Winter 1997, pp. 9–13, NAE, and P.A. DiMilla, K. Barbee, and D.A. Lauffenburger, "A Mathematical Model for the Effects of Adhesion and Mechanics on Cell Migration Speed," *Biophysics Journal* 60: 15–37 (1991).

[9] "The Emergence of Bioengineering," Robert M. Nerem, *The Bridge,* Volume 27, Number 4, Winter 1997, pp. 4–8, NAE.

[10] *The Whitaker Foundation Annual Report, 1997,* 1700 North Moore Street, Suite 2200, Rosslyn, VA 22209.

[11] "The AIMBE News," Volume 7, Issue 4, 1901 Pennsylvania Avenue, N.W., Suite 401, Washington, D.C.

Interorganizational cooperation and coordination among the various professionals engaged in medical device development will certainly advance device realization. The Center for Innovative Minimally Invasive Therapy (CIMIT), a consortium of the Massachusetts General Hospital, Brigham and Women's Hospital, Draper Laboratories, and Massachusetts Institute of Technology is one such example. CIMIT's goal is to combine clinical and technological resources in order to generate, develop, and reduce-to-practice innovative and high-impact concepts in minimally invasive therapy that improve the quality and lower the cost of health care delivery. A west coast counterpart is Stanford's Medical Device Network (MDN), which brings together physicians, engineers and scientists in the San Francisco Bay Area to encourage and facilitate invention, patenting, and early development of biomedical devices and instruments. A $150 million grant to Stanford from the founder of Netscape is intended to support MDN.

Biomedical device innovation—in terms of skilled and committed people, organization, and resources—has advanced significantly since the 1960s NAE-CIEBM efforts and the 1987 NAE-IOM study.

A REGULATORY PERSPECTIVE
David W. Feigal, Jr., M.D., M.P.H.
Director, Center for Devices and Radiological Health
Food and Drug Administration

Devices really span the entire culture of FDA because there are devices that are combined with drugs or biologics and there are biologics that are devices. The FDA Center for Drug Evaluation and Research (CDER) is driven by efficacy and exclusivity in drug development, as well as safety. The Center for Biologics Evaluation and Research (CBER), with more of a biotechnology focus than CDER, differs from the latter in that it has limited ability to confer exclusivity. All of FDA grapples with the definition of "biologics."

The Public Health Service Act has not been substantially modified since 1944; the existing definition does not even mention bacterial products. The Act says, "products analogous to viruses," and bacterial products are covered on that basis. With biological products, there is a tremendous sensitivity and fear of infectious diseases. Fear of infection is one of the challenges facing xenotransplantation, for example. However, the actual disease transmission rate with blood products today is lower than it has ever been.

One of the things that shapes the device industry is the fact that there is a wide diversity in risk. In addition, devices face the most detailed laws for therapeutics, down to minute specifications of some of the post-marketing features. Device law has authorities that do not exist for other products, such as true recall and product tracking.

The Center for Devices and Radiologic Health (CDRH), which regulates devices, has its cultural origins in responses to unsafe manufacturing practices of the past, false and misleading advertising, and fraud. To address manufacturing fraud, FDA developed good manufacturing practices, and for laboratory fraud it created good laboratory practices. Good clinical practice is one of the set of the regulations that involve Institutional Review Boards (IRBs), informed consent, record keeping, and ethical treatment of patients and research subjects. In addition, FDA has guidance for tissue screening, and even poor regulatory practice, turning the remedy upon itself to develop good review practices. In the recent past, FDA has made efforts to speed the approval process, responding to criticism from industry, Congress, and the public that it took too long. User fees placed stringent performance criteria not just on product review times but also on the review process itself.

An issue that reviewers and FDA take very seriously is the Food, Drug and Cosmetics Act requirement that a minimum level of quality of evidence is necessary to make some decisions. What is not at all intuitive to physicians is that the advertising standard for manufacturers having an approved claim is higher than that for the practice of medicine. That is why off-label medicine is allowed and physicians have to make choices.

FDA standards for biologics refer to safety, purity, and potency. Potency is a form of efficacy. Other standards require products to be unadulterated and not misbranded. Prior to 1962, devices were regulated as a drug. One device standard requires well-controlled investigations and other valid scientific evidence sufficient to determine effectiveness. That provides a lot of flexibility in the device area, more than exists in the drug standard. Devices explicitly face a risk-based standard, where the type of evidence depends on the classification of the devices. Humanitarian device exemptions are an example where the standard is changed for a specific area. Changes in technology have influenced FDA's view of product development. Sometimes the technology is embedded in the products themselves, for example, high-throughput screening, rational drug design, bioengineering, and miniaturization.

The culture of industry-FDA interactions has changed; there are more modular and agreement meetings and increased emphasis on determining least burdensome regulatory paths. Another aspect of regulatory change has been to put more emphasis on special populations, meeting the needs of children and the elderly, and making sure that women are adequately studied. Other changes in the process that have occurred include more transparency, harmonization with Europe and the Health Care Financing Administration (HCFA),[12] and responding to new laws. Increasingly complex communications exist among FDA, sponsors, manufacturers, research institutions, IRBs, trade associations, professional societies, third-party payers, and, in some cases, the Federal Trade Commission, depending on the nature of the product.

FDA is also seeing more complex conflict-of-interest situations, in which there may be an investigator-manufacturer-innovator with responsibilities to his or her university, or who may have Cooperative Research and Development

---

[12] Now Centers for Medicare and Medicaid Services (CMS).

Agreement with NIH. This person might also be the health professional who is taking care of the patient at the same time.

Another complex scenario for FDA occurs when a health facility becomes the manufacturer. In the setting of *in vitro* diagnostics, the local clinical laboratory might decide to develop a unique test (the regulatory nickname for this is "home brew"). FDA traditionally has stepped back from oversight in this area, in part because it could overwhelm its resources, and in part because the Clinical Laboratory Improvement Act provides some supervision of these laboratories. This is an especially hot topic in the area of genetic testing, where laboratories that have specialized in parts of the genome do not intend to become a manufacturer in the usual commercial sense. They will offer the test at one site. FDA still has jurisdiction over these facilities, but it challenges the old-fashioned paradigm in which a manufacturer is making a relatively limited number of products and shipping them nationwide. Another area receiving a lot of attention is the health facility that refurbishes single-use devices. They are manufacturers and thus are subject to FDA oversight.

It is crucial to remember that FDA was established at the time of Henry Ford's vision of the mass manufacturing of products, which assumed a standardized unit would be sold to everyone. Today, FDA increasingly faces individual products that are customized for the individual, just as customers get personalized coupons at the supermarket checkout based on a computer list of previous purchases.

Every business day, the device industry introduces 50 new products into the marketplace. Of those 50 new products, half are exempt from any type of premarket application. In 1998, CDRH reviewed over 4,500 applications. New drug applications and biologics license applications average between 2.5 and 5 man-years of review time. The amount of time and the resources that FDA dedicates to device approval is already quite low. There are about 900 different device types that FDA could write guidance about, given the proper resources.

One hundred years after the creation of FDA, the challenges are both the same and different. The Internet has replaced magazine ads as the home of the "patent nostrums." Interstate commerce has become international commerce. New products are still developed for mass markets by large corporations, but increasingly new products are tailored for small markets, sometimes even the individual patient. Eight thousand United States device manufacturers are joined by thousands of clinical laboratories and hospitals in developing custom diagnostics, implantables, and crafting new devices from tissue. Surgery and clinical pathology are blending into manufacturing. Instead of large manufacturers with few products, there are small manufacturers with thousands of variations on custom products. Mechanization, the great hope of the last century, has been replaced by information and the promise of genomics. Innovation and consumer protection are allies. Rapid change requires confidence and assurance of the integrity of the regulatory process.

AN INDUSTRY PERSPECTIVE: CHALLENGES IN THE DEVELOPMENT AND REGULATION OF DRUG-DEVICE COMBINATION PRODUCTS

Tobias Massa, Ph.D., DABT
Executive Director, Global Regulatory Affairs
Eli Lilly and Company

Pharmaceutical manufacturers have traditionally used devices for delivery of parenteral administration of drugs. In the United States, devices such as syringes and infusion pumps are approved by the FDA Center for Devices and Radiological Health (CDRH) as 510(k) applications. In more recent years, disposable and reusable devices for administration of drugs have been approved. These have offered the benefit of convenience and ease of use for patients faced with chronic (and in many cases lifetime) multiple daily injections. When sold together, these drug-device combination products are most often regulated and approved by the Center for Drug Evaluation and Research (CDER).

Drugs for the treatment of asthma, chronic obstructive pulmonary disease, and seasonal allergic rhinitis have made extensive use of metered dose inhalers (MDIs) and dry powder inhalers (DPIs). These represent true drug-device combination products that cannot be developed independently of one another because the dose administered to the patient is dependent on the drug and functional characteristics of the device. The use of MDIs and DPIs currently is expanding beyond the treatment of disorders limited to the respiratory system. Combination products for the systemic distribution of drugs such as insulin, parathyroid hormone (PTH), growth hormone, and other proteins utilizing pulmonary administration are under development. The advantages of inhalation as a route of administration, compared with parenteral administration, are obvious. It is anticipated that the use of the pulmonary route of administration will increase as the technology associated with these dosage forms improves and the issues surrounding their development and approval are addressed. Such drug-device combination products challenge the regulatory system's approach to review and approval.

Industry and health authorities readily admit that these products pose unique challenges. The dose given to the patient, and therefore the safety and efficacy of the product, is dependent not only on the formulation of the drug product, but also on the performance characteristics of the device. Together, these determine the emitted dose and particle size distribution, and hence the respirable dose given to the patient. One must therefore consider the "product" to be the formulation and the device, which would include the container, valve, actuator, and any associated protective packaging. Development and regulation of these products is complicated further by the variety of devices available. Each is unique and raises specific issues that must be addressed to regulate these products adequately.

Until recently, regulation of MDIs and DPIs occurred exclusively in CDER, as only products intended to treat respiratory disorders utilized these products. CDER acted as the primary reviewer of the investigational new drugs (IND) and new drug applications (NDA) associated with these products, with consultation from CDRH to insure that the device portion of the combination product was developed properly and met appropriate regulatory standards. Thus, a manufacturer had to address the concerns of more than one office within FDA.

Although MDIs were first introduced in the late 1950s, there still is no comprehensive, approved guidance for their development. Prior to November 1998, manufacturers obtained advice from FDA on a case-by-case basis for each product under development. Although not considered by industry to be directly applicable, manufacturers have been asked to comply with certain aspects of the Reviewer Guidance for Premarket Notification for Anesthesiology and Respiratory Therapy issued in 1993. This process for obtaining guidance was considered highly unsatisfactory, as manufacturers perceived that it resulted in inconsistent, arbitrary, and unnecessarily conservative regulation of these products. Furthermore, United States regulations seemed inconsistent with those of other regions, such as Europe. Thus, the challenge faced by regulators and industry is agreement on a harmonized guidance that provides for adequate and sufficient control to assure safety and efficacy while not being overly conservative.

In November 1998, FDA published "Guidance for Industry on Metered Dose Inhalers (MDI) and Dry Powder Inhaler (DPI) Drug Products: Chemistry, Manufacturing and Controls Documentation," the first comprehensive guidance for these complex dosage forms. The guidance represents a compilation of the advice given by the FDA Pulmonary Division over the past 10 years and is based on the agency's experience in reviewing numerous applications for these products.

Industry agrees with many of the points made in the draft guidance. MDIs and DPIs are complex products, and they require special controls not used for the development and manufacture of other dosage forms. There are a number of issues, however, about which there is significant disagreement. There is general industry consensus that a number of the specifications proposed in the draft appear to be overly restrictive and do not offer sufficient flexibility to cover the variety of devices currently approved or under development. Limits for some specifications appear to be inappropriately tight without sufficient scientific justification. Some of these requirements are unique to FDA for these products.

The draft guidance suggests a "one size fits all" approach to several significant specifications, notably particle size distribution and content uniformity (referred to as "dose uniformity" in the European Union [EU]). The United States requirements for content uniformity are highly prescriptive and apply to both MDIs and DPIs. They are based on assumptions about manufacturing and analytical capabilities rather than demonstration of safety and effectiveness. The dosage form must meet the criteria in the guidance relative to the dose claimed on the label, and there is no provision for analysis of outlier test results. The EU guidance takes a more rational approach and suggests that the specification should be based on the data from material that was found to be safe and effective in clinical studies and on a reasonable assessment of potential variability in manufacturing capability and analytical methods. The United States requirements punish manufacturers who have the ability to control and monitor the manufacturing process carefully. The approach proposed in the draft FDA guidance is inconsistent with the principles for setting specifications in the International Conference on Harmonisation of Technical Requirements for Registration of Pharmaceuticals for Human Use (ICH) guidance Q6A.

The FDA guidance recommends specifications for spray pattern and extractable profiles. Neither of these is required in the EU guidance for DPIs. The FDA has suggested that spray pattern is an essential quality control parameter to assess valve and actuator function of MDIs. Specifications for size and shape of the spray pattern are recommended. It is acknowledged that one would not want the product emitted from the device to be presented to the patient in a narrow stream that would not allow proper inhalation of the dose. However, it has not been demonstrated that changes or differences in spray pattern are medically relevant; therefore, setting a tight specification for this parameter appears inappropriate. It has been suggested that this be addressed in development and correlated to dimensions of the device (valve and or actuator) that can be measured as a quality control test. If a specification cannot be avoided, a qualitative limit test might be more appropriate unless a quantitative limit can be scientifically justified by FDA.

The requirement for extractable profiles is also of concern. FDA has recommended that the elastomeric components of MDIs and DPIs undergo extraction in a number of different solvents to determine whether any constituents of the components can be extracted or leached by the solvents. The "fingerprint" of the extractables is expected to serve as a QC release test to insure that the supplier of the components has not made any changes in the composition of the constituent materials. It has also been stated that this test is required to insure patient safety. There are many objections to this line of thinking. First, many of the components are not in contact with the formulated drug, or are in contact with the formulation for very short periods of time upon actuation of the device during dosing. The amount of any potential extractables would be small relative to what could be found in a simulated extraction study. This test has little relevance for DPIs, which do not contain any solvents. Lastly, the amount of material extracted in such studies is rarely found to be at toxicologically relevant levels. Industry has suggested that this test is appropriate for use in development of MDIs to determine whether any potentially toxic extractables are present at levels that might be of concern. There appears to be lack of sufficient scientific justification for this requirement as a routine quality control test. The draft guidance also requires determination of stability under a number of conditions that go beyond the ICH stability guidance Q1A.

Companies developing pulmonary dosage forms are frequently asked to comply with certain requirements in the CDRH Guidance for Premarket Notification Submission. This guidance is written to regulate devices intended for use in operating rooms and hospital settings. It was not written with consideration of drug device combination products. For example, these products are expected to pass a fluid spill resistance test, also known as drip testing. The test involves pouring a large quantity of water over the device, after which the device is expected to meet its functional release testing. It is hard to imagine why this test should apply to dry powder inhalers. It seems much more appropriate to label these products with a warning to keep them away from wet environments. The CDRH guidance also prescribes temperature, pressure, and humidity extremes under which mechanical performance must be demonstrated. Such extremes are not specified in EU guidance for DPIs.

The draft FDA guidance also prescribes extremely tight specification for impurities in propellants used in MDIs. These limits were developed based on process and analytical capabilities of the propellant suppliers, not on toxicological assessment. In many cases, the limits are thousands of times lower than the no-effect toxicological limits for the impurities in question and are much tighter than current compendial limits. Given that these propellants have been used for many years in MDIs, one must ask why the limits have been set so low. FDA has stated that the tight limits are necessary due to the issues surrounding the short supply of CFC propellants (due to the phase out of these materials per the Montreal Protocol) and their concerns with stockpiling, recycling, and illegal importation. While these concerns may be valid, the tight limits appear to penalize manufacturers who adhere to regulations and guidance. A more appropriate method to deal with such concerns might be to provide severe penalties for violation of such regulations if they are indeed such a threat to public health.

The most difficult provision in the FDA draft guidance is the requirement that the commercial drug device combination be used in pivotal clinical trials to determine safety and efficacy. FDA strongly advises against changes to the device once the pivotal clinical and stability studies are initiated. When combined with the requirement for 2-year safety studies of products such as insulin and PTH, the use of the final commercial product in these trials is a significant issue for manufacturers. It requires that commercial development be completed long before the product has been shown to be safe and effective and therefore commercially viable. This policy also creates a system in which device optimization may not occur until after product approval due to severely compressed time lines to have a commercial product by Phase 3. Unlike drugs given by other routes of administration, there is no provision to conduct bridging bioequivalence studies for pulmonary combination products. FDA has stated that it is difficult, if not impossible, to demonstrate the bioequivalence of products delivered using pulmonary administration. This position has resulted from their experience with devices used to treat asthma and COPD. The low doses of the steroids and beta-blockers used in these products make determination of blood levels virtually impossible. The sponsors must rely on clinical trials using pulmonary function tests to demonstrate equivalence. This is difficult at best, as evidenced by the paucity of generic oral and nasal inhalation products. However, this situation might be different for some of the protein products currently under development, such as insulin, PTH, and growth hormone, which may have adequate surrogate markers to allow for determination of bioequivalence. The guidance should allow sufficient flexibility to accommodate this possibility.

It is clearly recognized by industry that these products are unique, in that the dose seen by the patient is dependent on the formulation and the performance characteristics of the device. They require equally unique specifications to ensure that a defined dose can be administered reproducibly to the patient and that the combination product is safe and effective in patient use. There is a need to balance setting reasonable product specifications with protection of public health and safety. The current system will continue to result in specifications being set unreasonably, resulting in batches of product being rejected at release or failing on stability unnecessarily. Harmonization of United States requirements with those of other regions, particularly the EU, is also necessary to insure adequate utilization of resources and avoid unnecessary clinical and *in vitro* testing.

AN EVALUATOR'S PERSPECTIVE
Joel J. Nobel, M.D.
President, ECRI
and
Jeffrey C. Lerner, Ph.D.
Vice President for Strategic Planning, ECRI

Clinical acceptance of new medical devices, drugs, or biotechnologies and overcoming the hurdles of coverage and payment reimbursements depends heavily on the results of clinical trials and technology assessment. ECRI (formerly the Emergency Care Research Institute) is a non-profit health services research organization that for 30 years has evaluated a wide range of medical products, ranging from complex imaging systems to anti-needle stick devices and blood chemistry analyzers and critical care monitors to surgical gloves. ECRI's technology assessment program focuses more broadly on drugs, devices, biotechnologies, and medical and surgical procedures, examining efficacy, safety, cost-effectiveness, and, in some cases, ethical and legal issues associated with a specific technology. While ECRI operates at financial arm's length from industry, it also works closely with industry to resolve differences in views, resolve hazards, and improve products, and for the most part, in a climate of mutual respect.

Clinical trials data is a critical element in evaluation or assessment, regulation, or reimbursement, and so ECRI has about 30 years of experience in examining peer review clinical studies, most of which have emerged from academic institutions, and ECRI examines these studies in a way that is far tougher than the original peer review process. Most peer-reviewed journal articles emerging from the academic medical community simply will not support evidence-based medicine. They do not provide evidence to support decisions about what works, how well it works, and whether or not it is worth doing.

The first step in technology assessment is to collect information on all that is known about a technology. Typically, less than 5% of peer-reviewed journal articles in oncology or surgery can withstand serious scrutiny and stand up well over the years. It is a bit better in the cardiovascular literature. Financial, psychological, career, or other incentives can distort the process. In addition, responsibility for clinical research is too diffuse. While this has certain values, it also dilutes responsibility and in doing so makes accountability hard to pinpoint. Even when clinical studies do get it right, the results are often ignored. Electronic fetal monitoring has been repeatedly shown to have little benefit, yet it is ubiquitous.

Another factor is that research in academic centers is not adequately managed. An academic institution produces many intellectual products and some patented physical products, but it lacks any analogue of a quality control manager typical of industry or research laboratories. Academic institutions lack requirements for basic elements like retention time for research records, control of laboratory notebooks, back-up requirements for computer data, data auditing, or any core quality measures typical of most other types of institutions doing research or producing goods.

Research funding sources and funding relationships distort motivation, method, thought processes, results, and presentation. And, whatever its virtues, maintaining the value of academic freedom takes precedence over any type of institutional oversight and responsibility for the quality of research.

Clinical research today deserves examination and reform at a fundamental structural level. Disclosure of research funding sources is essential. The disclosure certification has to ask questions in a very thoughtful way because many types of remuneration have been designed to be concealed. Clinical research needs a code of ethics to which investigators should make a contractual commitment, preferably one with penalties for violation. Clinical research in academic institutions desperately needs ongoing quality management to improve the quality of the studies undertaken by the majority of researchers who are honest.

INNOVATION AND INVENTION IN MEDICAL DEVICES: IMPLANTABLE DEFIBRILLATORS
Glen D. Nelson, M.D.
Vice Chair, Medtronic, Inc.

Approximately 25 million Americans today benefit from therapeutic implants. Because of the site-specific nature of device therapies and method of action, there are few, if any, metabolic side effects or interactions. In contrast to pharmaceuticals, implants are typically immune from patient compliance problems. This holds implications for the overall quality of outcomes for individual patients and patient populations and more easily allows researchers to measure the results.

Implants are indicated only when simpler therapeutic alternatives do not exist or are markedly less effective. For example, an NIH-sponsored, multicenter, unsustained tachycardia trial clarified the risk of sudden cardiac death in certain patients who had suffered a previous myocardial infarction. The risk of sudden death was found to be 32% at 5 years for patients who had a history of coronary heart disease, decreased heart function, and short episodes of nonsustained ventricular tachycardia, even if frontline medications were administered.[13] In contrast, susceptible patients who received an implanted cardiodefibrillator exhibited a 74% reduction in sudden cardiac death compared with those patients receiving medications only. According to the study, if the findings were applied in clinical practice, up to 65,000 lives would be saved.[14]

Reimbursement for such devices continues to be a significant barrier. Provisional coverage following FDA approval or clearance for PMA devices will speed the availability of technology when it has real value. A secondary effect of reimbursement pressures is a reduction in the amount of public financing available to small start-up companies. This has a restrictive effect on researchers' ability to develop leading-edge technology. Cost-containment pressure focuses on event costs, and fails to assess the relative comprehensive costs of therapeutic alternatives over the entire course of the disease and over a patient's life.

Economic models are not well developed, so focusing on the event costs leads to the view that technology is the culprit in health care cost escalation. Economic models tend to ignore broader social and economic benefits as patients return to self-reliance and family members or caregivers are relieved of their support roles. In addition, fear of litigation has often limited researchers' ability as manufacturers to produce new technology because material manufacturers are afraid of the litigious circumstances.

Medical devices are often mistakenly perceived to follow the pharmaceutical model. Unlike pharmaceuticals—where therapeutic formulation remains essentially unchanged for the commercial lifetime of the agent—medical device technologies undergo continual and progressive evolutionary improvement. For example, defibrillators were developed over a period of 10 years at Medtronic, yielding a series of improvements in the basic device. The most striking improvement is significant size reduction, a result of breakthroughs in power sources, microelectronics, new capacitors, and packaging technology. Size is important to patient comfort. Achieving smaller size without sacrificing capability also reduces the potential for certain complications, including erosion of the implant, which is particularly important in slender people or children. What is even more clinically significant is that device longevity has been extended by years from those first generations from 2 or 3, to 10 or 12 years. Breakthroughs in defibrillation stimulation patterns and lead technology have removed the requirement for opening the chest to implant the leads to use these devices, resulting in a five-fold reduction in the mortality risk of the procedure. Arrhythmia detection algorithms have been enhanced to minimize false positives and negatives. Detection and stimulation advances have led to therapies that can block

---

[13] "A Randomized Study of the Prevention of Sudden Death in Patients with Coronary Artery Disease," Alfred E. Buxton, Kerry L. Lee, John D. Fisher, Mark E. Josephson, Eric N. Prystowsky, and Gail Hafley, *The New England Journal of Medicine,* Volume 341, Number 25, 1999, pp. 1882–1890.

[14] "Prophylactic Implantable Cardioverter Defibrillator Trials: MUSTT, MADIT, and Beyond," Eric N. Prystowsky and Seah Nisam, *The American Journal of Cardiology,* Volume 86, 2000, pp. 1214–1215.

the emergence of the most serious arrhythmias and ventricular afibrillation and literally overpace the arrhythmias before you get to the end stage of having to deliver a shock. Finally, onboard EKG storage capabilities provide cardiologists with important information on rhythm detection, therapy effectiveness, and help to guide the ongoing therapy. Figure 1 illustrates how cost-effectiveness for medical devices typically increases with subsequent device generation.

The first generations of implantable defibrillators were marginally cost-effective. Within a few years, cost-effectiveness improved substantially as a result of lower power microelectronics and advances in power source energy capacity. The advances extended the lifetime service of the defibrillators and delayed markedly the need for replacement devices and the attendant costs. Advances in lead technology and stimulation patterns in the 1990s made practical the implantation of these devices via a transvenous route.

Interestingly, although the event costs of implantation are substantial (estimated at around $45,000, including the cost of the devices and the hospitalization), some studies suggest that the current technology generations represent cost savings versus the alternatives, and that is a difficult analysis because often the endpoint with this particular device is death. This cost reduction is the result of continual improvements in efficacy brought about by progressive advances in

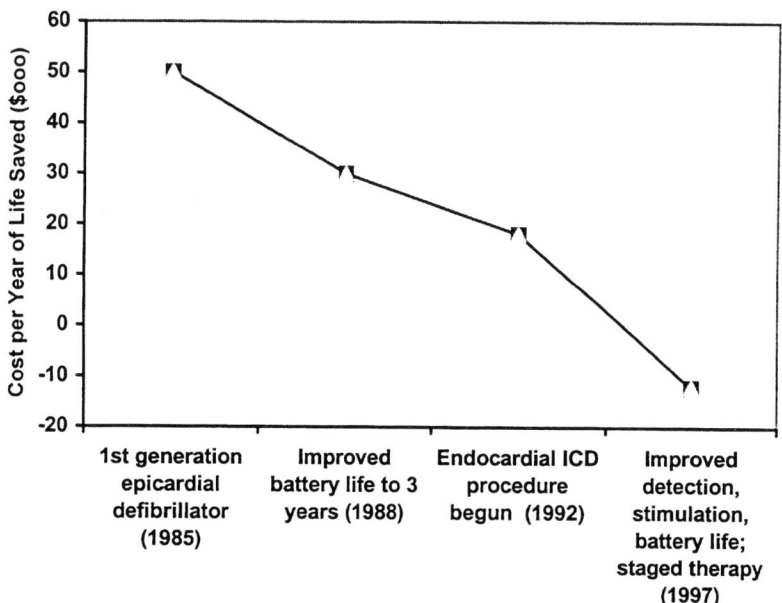

FIGURE 1 The impact of technological evolution on cost-effectiveness of implantable cardioverter-defibrillator.

arrhythmia detection and stimulation algorithms and further extensions of battery life, and also because of the multifunctional capabilities of today's devices that permit them to adapt automatically to changes in the patient's clinical and physiologic status.

These technological advances, in combination, have markedly reduced unplanned hospitalizations as well as dependence on costly concomitant medical treatments. While this example relates specifically to implantable pulse defibrillators, the pattern of progressive cost-effectiveness and improvement resulting from next generational technological and technique advances is a hallmark for essentially all medical device technology. Thus, each new generation is almost invariably more cost-effective than its predecessor.

Patients derive demonstrable benefit from a process that encourages the prompt introduction of the next generations of medical devices. These benefits include substantial reductions in morbidity and mortality, enhanced efficacy, fewer complications, and greater transparency between the normal condition and the treated circumstance.

Researchers will continue to see value-added advances in medical device therapies that are currently serving patients. These devices will approximate lost natural function and exhibit intrinsic capabilities that will allow them to automatically adapt to changes in the underlying condition of the patient. Devices will become more biological. Prosthetic heart valves for instance, will probably possess physical and mechanical characteristics that will permit them to be implanted when they are needed to replace natural valves that have become incompetent. In addition to acting as valves, they will serve as substrates for the attraction, differentiation, and ingrowth of living cells that over a period of time will replace the synthetic structures implanted. In time, these tissue-engineered structures will be indistinguishable from normal natural tissue. Such approaches are already entering the clinical setting in the form of skin substitutes and replacement for bone, ligaments, and cartilage.

Combination devices that deliver gene therapies to specific sites of interest and for required periods of time are another way that devices will progressively become more biological. Such approaches offer the distinct possibility of disease cures rather than palliative treatments, as is now the case. Although researchers are naturally attracted to the exciting possibilities of emerging and future therapeutic medical devices, the area of implanted diagnostics and monitoring holds enormous potential.

Next generations of technology will literally close the loop on therapy. The implantable monitor, for example, will continually be vigilant to the patient's circumstances, and when something serious occurs, appropriate words can be sent by telemetry or the device itself can automatically respond just as the defibrillator does when it detects some abnormal rhythm that will lead to ventricular fibrillation. In some cases, as with a low battery indicator, the alert will be sent only to the patient, so he or she can have the device checked. This scenario presents a dramatic application of monitoring capabilities, and the most clinically relevant contributions will be in quality improvement aspects.

Patient compliance, however, remains a serious limitation in chronic disease treatment. Implantable monitoring will likely provide much better guidance as to when treatments are suboptimal due to the regimen selected or due to a failure to follow prescribed drug administration protocols. Chronic monitoring will permit physicians to match treatment options more closely to the patient's abilities, thereby improving overall quality. The convergence of traditional medical technology with communication and Internet technology presents a remarkable opportunity to change the face of health care.

Dramatic quality improvements can result from consistent application of statistically based medical care algorithms based on broad and deep databases. Real-time access of these large databases will identify trends so that the health care system can be more dynamic and at the same time knowledge-based, and perhaps far less dependent on small clinical trials. Using databases that are automatically generated by automatic acquisition from devices, combined with caregivers' databases, will allow researchers to apply deep computing approaches to identify trends early and to create optimal treatment algorithms.

GENERAL DISCUSSION OF THE KEYNOTE SESSION

John Watson of NIH began the discussion by inquiring about the Product Quality Research Institute (PQRI). Tobias Massa from Eli Lilly described the new institute as the brainchild of Roger Williams, whose grand design has industry, academia, and government coming together to try to address common quality issues associated with pharmaceutical products. Funded by pharmaceutical corporations and trade organizations, PQRI currently sponsors four technical committees dealing in the areas of drug substance, drug product, biopharmaceutics (issues related to bioequivalence), and science management, which is seeking to map the regulatory review process. According to Dr. Massa, working groups are looking at specific questions related to those four areas, for example, blend uniformity analysis. That is, what is the best way to assure content uniformity of products? Some of these projects will be carried out at FDA, and some will be carried out at individual companies volunteering to do this work in their own laboratories.

Clifford Goodman then returned to Glen Nelson's remarks on the challenge of demonstrating cost-effectiveness, pointing out that many devices that Nelson's company makes call for a substantial initial expense, between hardware and implant surgery, and do not start saving money until later. So, there is a time factor in considering cost-effectiveness. Furthermore, he noted, Nelson's cost-effectiveness data did not even mention productivity, that is the averted costs of lost productivity, something else difficult to quantify because it does not start saving money immediately, nor do researchers generally capture the financial savings from letting people stay at work. Goodman brought up the case of the HMO that loses 15 percent of its enrollees every year and therefore might not care about long-range savings from use of an expensive device because the patient will probably not be enrolled long enough to recoup the investment. He then asked the group for their thoughts on whether the inability or unwillingness of such payers is in fact affecting decisions about which technologies to undertake and build.

Dr. Nelson replied that it definitely affects innovation, and drew on his experience as a managed care company director to describe a proposal to reduce the sort of disincentive that Dr. Goodman cited, namely a surcharge that would make funding available for long-term interventions that do not have to be driven by a 1-year actuarial mentality. Unanswered questions include who is given responsibility for administering that fund and whether it would allow for earlier reimbursement for therapies that not only are promising now, but are bound to become dramatically cost-effective in the societal sense after a couple of revisions. Nelson also reinforced Goodman's complaint that researchers need economic models that include a method of assigning a value to the fact that not only patients but also spouses or other caregivers can go back to work after an expensive intervention like an implant. These outcomes, he asserted, are not only heartwarming, but also have huge economic impacts that vastly outweigh the cost of the device. Where do you recognize those savings, he asked, and how do you channel them back then into the further development of that technology?

Ron Geigle, from the consulting firm Polidais, offered the observation that in the policy world of Washington there is a growing disconnect between the nature of evidence that is appropriate for devices and the nature of evidence that is appropriate for drugs. That is, he said, one can see a growing tendency to insist upon randomized controlled clinical trials as the gold standard, and yet this morning a lot was said about exciting technologies, technologies that are changing rapidly, nanotechnologies, information technologies, Internet-connected-to-patient monitoring, closed-loop systems, quick half-lives. Geigle's questions for Dr. Nelson and the group were whether there are assessment models that work best for those sorts of technologies, and secondly, what is the effect of the imposition of randomized controlled clinical trials on that kind of device-innovation process and the capacity of companies to innovate and attract venture capital? How do researchers create an understanding in Washington that devices are different from drugs and ought to be evaluated with a different model of evidence?

Dr. Nelson agreed with Dr. Geigle's articulation of the problem, pointing out that the major R&D costs for companies like his are in the clinical trial phase, where it is extremely difficult to randomize and use sham procedures. He noted that trials seem to have scientific rigor, but are costly, and in his view are not beneficial. Instead, he argued, postmarket surveillance is one means of reducing those costs and maybe at the same time improving the outcomes. Devices or pharmaceuticals or surgical procedures will never be perfect; researchers and practitioners must learn as quickly as possible whether there are imperfections that can be corrected. Nelson pointed out that no one wants to go back to the era where irradiating the thymus gland of children resulted in thyroid cancer 20 years later, but, by the same token, open heart surgery in the 50s led to a mortality rate of 50 percent for ventricular septal defects. There are no reimbursers in the United States or the world today that would pay for a procedure with those statistics. Yet the current mortality rate for a ventricular septal defect repair is probably about 0.3 percent. The point, according to Dr. Nelson, is that researchers have to move through these periods of potential poor medical results to get to better medical results. He offered the example of Charles Bailey, who lost five patients in a row fracturing mitral valves and lost his privileges at every hospital in Philadelphia, but when he did the sixth, and it was successful, it opened a whole new field of surgery. Nelson confessed he does not know how to draw the line, but feels it is important to accept some lesser level of performance knowing that later iterations will not only be cost-effective but will be enormously valuable in terms of people's quality of life.

Dr. Nobel replied that he certainly agrees with the proposition that randomized controlled trials are not appropriate for certain types of medical products, and that presents an education problem for the people who provide reimbursement. It is not a reasonable gold standard, he said, and is not even applicable in many cases. It is thoroughly impractical and in some cases plainly unethical to do certain types of studies, but he noted that it is natural for a large government reimburser, or even a large private one, to want to have a simplified rule book. It makes life easy, but the diversity of medical devices requires a diversity of proving methods, and that is an intellectual and educational challenge for the people in this group and people who pay for patient care.

David Feigal from the FDA offered some thoughts on the reimbursement decisions facing HCFA, noting that they have different criteria for reimbursement, one of which is value added, something that is not required for drug approval or device approval by FDA. There are countries in Europe that have a comparative claims requirement. That is, they require comparison of the new product relative to the existing products that they resemble, but that has never been the standard in the United States. Third-party payers often want just that sort of data. This is an area where knowing the rules may help the process because of the opportunity during development to consider whether collecting that comparative data is desirable, even if it is not necessary for FDA approval.

Dr. Feigal also felt that the rapid evolution of devices often makes it unclear what it is that HCFA is agreeing to reimburse. That is, if they approve a pacemaker today, and 3 or 4 years later the manufacturer has a new-generation product, a totally different device, will they revisit that decision or are accept the fact that they already thought through this general category? If the former, does that create incentives not to innovate and to leave things frozen so that people do not lose the reimbursement approval? From FDA's standpoint it might have been an incremental change that would have been quite acceptable, but given the limited data set available to the third party reimburser, it may well trigger the response, "We need to have some clinical evidence."

Feigal's final comment was to remind the group that even for drugs the definition of adequate and well-controlled trials lists five examples, only one of which is the randomized double-blind placebo-controlled trial. The historical control is another, at the other extreme. In between are dose-response, no-treatment control, and active control, and you can find approvals that use each of the different types of evidence. So, he averred, researchers need to ask in every case, "What are we trying to learn, and what are the difficulties with the evidence in this field?" He gave an example from a recent review of cardiac therapy during which an FDA reviewer pointed to the restenosis rates of the control groups of five randomized controlled trials and said, "They have to do more randomized controlled trials because the control groups vary between 5 percent and 30 percent, which is exactly the same range, maybe a bit higher, as the benefit groups." But whenever there was a direct comparison there always was a benefit! There is not going to be a single answer for this, he concluded, but these are science- and evidence-based decisions, and they require exactly the kind of information clinicians want in making decisions for their patients. Neither they nor FDA want or need overkill.

Jim Benson with the Health Industry Manufacturers Association (HIMA) [Editor's note: now Advanced Medical Technology Association (AdvaMed)] then returned to an earlier point and asked the group to think about who pays the bills: in the case of HCFA reimbursement, the taxpayers, and in the case of HMOs and other private insurers, the employers. All of it comes out of the worker's salary in one form or another, yet, he said, researchers do not seem to target their studies and their research toward the benefit that goes to those two communities, the taxpayers and the employers that are paying the HMOs. Maybe the industrial community and others really need to include that in some of their cost-effectiveness work and really aim at convincing not HCFA, which does not really have any choice, but the taxpayers and employers, that some of this innovation can actually save money.

Dr. Nelson agreed that consumers are going to have a lot larger role in determining their health care, and their view of value may be a lot different than the view of their managed care organizations. He pointed out that the problem with just appealing to the individual consumer is that the natural response is to abandon the original spending accounts and let everybody just spend their own money on health care. But, he said, researchers really do need an insurance mentality that takes care of the individual whose costs will be 100 times the average. People have accepted as a society that they are going to amalgamate their risk, although there are lots of things working against it. People cannot pull the bottom can out of a grocery store display and do away with insurance.

Dr. Mann extended the discussion by drawing on his experience chairing a National Academy of Sciences conference on technology to aid the blind that made two points. One was that the federal government at that time was spending on the order of $10 to $100 per cancer and cardiac victim and $.02 per blind person, and the other part was that if one made a blind person a taxpayer through reading access and mobility one was, in fact, being very cost-effective. The second point was that a lot of the work at MIT on the "Boston Arm" prosthesis was funded in part by the Liberty Mutual Insurance Company. As an insurance company writing worker's compensation policies it was to their financial advantage to be able not only to advertise that they were doing great things for humanity but also to show that they were reducing their rehabilitation costs by providing a better prosthesis.

Tom Loarie, CEO of Kera Vision Inc., had the last word in the morning's discussion, using personal experience to illustrate the point that assessing new technologies at the very early stages of development is very difficult, even for sophisticated people in the business. As a young engineer at a company called American Hospital Supply Corporation, he witnessed the company looking into acquiring a small firm making a pacemaker. In those days it was probably a $30 million to $40 million business, and they came back and said, "You know, that is really not going to amount to much." American Hospital Supply does not exist anymore, but Medtronic does.

Loarie's second point was his belief that the crux of the problem is that in this and other western countries researchers like to believe that everyone should have equal access to new technology. He asked the group to imagine if researchers had decided in the early 1980s that the car phone was something every citizen of this country should be required to have, or simply have a right to, at $3,000 per unit. A car phone is very much like a medical device, he asserted. It is engineering-based. It goes through the iterative process and as researchers learn, as they improve it, they reduce costs, and the market eventually expands. It is, however, very different from a drug, in that it is introduced into the market at the very highest point in its cost. Researchers face this dilemma of providing it to the masses, while government steadily adds to the cost. He argued that these conflicting demands build in a tremendous prejudice against the approval of new technologies, and it is the only part of this economy where technology is looked at as a scapegoat.

3
The Nature of Medical Innovation

Presentations in this session of the Workshop provided background and context for the status of innovation in medical devices since the late 1980s, and addressed the invention and development process map for medical device technologies and products. Several case studies were offered to analyze the factors that have led to significant medical device innovations in the past 50 years. Speakers discussed the factors that have supported significant ongoing and emerging technology innovations to reach the development and clinical stage.[1]

THE INNOVATIVE PROCESS FOR MEDICAL DEVICES: A NASA PERSPECTIVE
John Hines, M.S.
Technology Development Manager
Space Life Sciences Program
and
Joan Vernikos, Ph.D.
Director, Life Sciences Division
National Aeronautics and Space Administration

Since its inception in 1958, NASA has collaborated with many entities on technology R&D. These collaborations have included the development of medical devices in support of astronaut health and biomedical research, both on the

---

[1] One presenter, Dean Kamen, President of DEKA Research and Development Corporation, played a videotape from a news show that aired on network television.

ground and in space. This collaborative R&D process has been based on the need to utilize a broad range of expertise and experience to meet special requirements, minimize development costs, and exercise the NASA mandate to "provide for the widest practicable ... dissemination of information concerning its activities and the results thereof."

From the earliest years of the United States Space Program, NASA has in many cases taken off-the-shelf commercial biomedical instruments and modified them for use in space. This process mainly involved the use of NASA customized components and packaging designed to survive the rigors of space flight, and special considerations for safety and materials composition. NASA's special requirements overlapped to a significant extent with military requirements for biomedical devices, including several core needs: portability, operation within intravehicular and extravehicular environments, telecommunication of data, minimally invasive sensors and non-encumbering instrumentation, and low-power, 28VDC and/or battery-powered systems.

NASA has always had especially challenging requirements for medical devices, including operation in variable pressure environments (space capsules and space suits), high radiation environments, and high vibration and shock environments (launch/reentry). Paramount in these considerations for medical devices has been the safety and well being of the astronaut crew and biological subjects. To this end, devices have been designed with the highest medical device standards in mind, and rigorous testing has been performed to validate their performance. In addition, NASA has high reliability requirements for biomedical devices, since on-orbit repair and/or replacement often is not possible. Some of these requirements overlap in part with those of the emergency medical monitoring and transport industry.

More recently, NASA's Life Sciences Division has established internal Advanced Technology Development (ATD) programs to anticipate needs for medical (and biological) devices and similar technology. Because it can take years to go from initial requirements to having flight-qualified hardware, one aim of the ATD-Biosensors Program has been to collaborate with the future users of biomedical technology and develop and demonstrate modular, prototype systems in anticipation of need. When requirements are more solidly defined, often by multiple users who need similar technology, these prototype systems can be more quickly assembled, tested, and made available for use.

NASA also has established multi-disciplinary teams to plan for integration of advanced technologies into the International Space Station (ISS). The ISS provides a special challenge for development of medical devices, as it is a large, international research laboratory built in space to remain for 10 to 15 years. Over that time period, medical technologies will rapidly evolve, and older technology will need to be infused with new modular systems that take advantage of industry-developed technologies to optimize functional performance at minimum cost. These include sensors and instrumentation, analytical tools, and specialty devices. The emerging medical device industry/academic focus on wireless, telemetric, wearable, automated, "intelligent assistant," reconfigurable technology fits well with NASA's needs for the future. The complementary emerging technologies of nanotechnology and biotechnology can greatly facilitate in-flight clinical analyses, and are also of great interest to NASA, due to their small size, low-power, low-cost disposable, and customizable features.

Medical Device Case Studies

NASA's transfer of its R&D results to the private sector has been implemented through various methods and mechanisms that provide industry and academia access to spin-off technologies and knowledge, several of which have been applied to commercial biomedical devices. This collaboration is enabled by the provisions of the Space Act Agreement, and is implemented with the assistance of the NASA Commercial Technology Offices (CTOs) by way of a variety of arrangements, including cooperative agreements, reimbursable and non-reimbursable space act agreements, memoranda of agreements, and inter-agency agreements. Additionally, NASA often develops requirements for new biomedical devices that are contracted out to industry or academia for R&D, with encouragement to industry to consider commercial development of the technology, when appropriate. On occasion, NASA biomedical technology developers have left government service to privately develop commercial versions of the technology they helped invent within the Agency. In these cases there has been both a knowledge and technology NASA spin-off.

Modification of commercial technology is an option whose practicality is assessed prior to initiating internal R&D. The dual-use and co-development of technology by NASA and other government or private-sector partners is a relatively new but expanding method for technology development, with biomedical devices being attractive candidates. For most medical device development funding is provided by NASA's Life Sciences Division. However, several medical device technologies developed by industry for the private sector have included technology components (and software) developed within NASA for non-life-sciences research, such as a smart probe for breast cancer diagnosis and treatment and a robotic neurosurgical device. Some examples of biomedical devices that illustrate these NASA Invention and Innovation process categories are described in the following sections.

Cardiac Monitor

A traditional method of assessing heart function is thermo-dilution, which involves the insertion of a catheter into a pulmonary artery. NASA needed a non-invasive system to monitor astronauts in flight. In 1965, Johnson Space Center contracted with the University of Minnesota to explore the concept of Impedance Cardiography (ICG). This led to the development of the Minnesota Impedance Cardiograph (MIC), an electronic system for measuring impedance changes across the thorax that would be reflective of cardiac function and blood flow from the left ventricle into the aorta. NASA separately contracted with Space Labs, Inc., for construction of space-qualified miniaturized impedance units based on the MIC technology. The system was introduced into service aboard Space Shuttle flight STS-8 in 1983. The ICG had potential for hospital applications, but further development was needed. A number of research institutions and medical equipment companies launched development of their own ICGs, using the MIC technology as a departure point.

Heart Imaging System

Doctors on the ground need to be able to evaluate the vital signs of astronauts in orbit. NASA has therefore researched and developed sophisticated heart monitoring systems for this purpose. Dr. Jeffrey L. Lacy was a biomedical researcher at Johnson Space Center who developed technology that was later adapted for commercial medical use. His research into heart imaging led to the development of the MultiWire Gamma Camera (MWGC), marketed by Xenos Medical Systems. This imaging system is six times faster than other devices, portable, and provides extremely high-resolution images. One of the key components of this system is its use of the radioisotope Tantalum-178 (Ta-178), which can be optimally imaged only with the MWGC. Use of Ta-178 has a major benefit: its short half-life means that it is only in the body for 9 minutes, while other radioisotopes must remain in a patient's system for 6 to 72 hours. Thus, Ta-178 provides a 20 to 200% decrease in radiation exposure during the imaging process. Since astronauts are exposed to chronic, low-level radiation during space flight, this reduced exposure is an especially important advantage for NASA.

Heart Assist Pump

The concept of a heart pump containing NASA technology began with talks between Dr. Michael DeBakey from the Baylor College of Medicine and NASA engineer David Saucier, who happened to one of Dr. DeBakey's heart transplant patients. Saucier felt compelled to help develop a device to assist the 30,000 people a year who are unable to obtain a donor heart, and he understood the Space Shuttle technology that could be applied to create an effective heart pump. Mechanical heart pumps have three potential problems: destruction of red blood cells, formation of blood clots, and the body's reaction to a more continuous blood flow rather than the normal pulsed flow of blood. A team from NASA Johnson Space Center and NASA Ames Research Center assisted Dr. DeBakey and his Baylor partners in the development of an effective heart pump by using super computers to analyze how shuttle fuel-flow dynamics could be used to reduce red cell damage to acceptable limits. This improved flow pattern also reduces the tendency for blood clots to form. The pump design was eventually licensed to MicroMed, which successfully ran clinical trials of the device in Europe. Efforts are underway to facilitate use of this device in the United States.

Telemedicine Instrumentation Pack

During space missions, NASA's astronauts are out of physical reach for doctors and surgeons on Earth. If an astronaut-physician is available onboard a spacecraft, ground-based remote monitoring medical support is essential to augment that available in-flight. Technology had to be developed to give flight surgeons at Mission Control the capability to conference with, diagnose, and treat astronauts in flight. NASA's intensive research into these systems led to the creation of new telemedicine instrumentation systems. The latest result of NASA's research into this field is the Telemedicine Instrumentation Pack (TIP), manufactured under contract to NASA by KRUG Life Sciences of Houston, Texas. Developed at Johnson Space Center, the TIP weighs about 25 pounds and is the size of a small suitcase. Designed to record and display video, audio, and biomedical data (such as ECG waveforms, heart rate, and blood pressure) the TIP allows a doctor to make accurate remote diagnoses. Advanced features still in development will include electronic medical information and literature, decision support systems, and computerized patient records.

Pill Telemetry Technologies

NASA contracted with Konigsberg Instruments in the 1970s to develop pill-type, implantable, multi-channel biotelemetry systems for animal research studies in space, and later an ingestible pill for human studies. In parallel, NASA, by way of a Goddard telemetry program, contracted with the Advanced Physics Lab (APL) at Johns Hopkins to develop an ingestible, temperature-sensing pill for health care applications. There was a direct spin-off of these technologies for battlefield biomedical monitoring by DoD during Operation Desert Storm, resulting in use of both the APL and Konigsberg ingestible pills. Also in the 1990s, the Sensors 2000! Advanced Technology Development program at NASA Ames Research Center developed a pill implant for pH and pressure monitoring during fetal surgery, which can also have applications to small animal research (mice) on the International Space Station.

Benefits of the NASA Process

NASA R&D in medical devices during the 1960s and 1970s typically included "contracting out" much of the development work to industry and/or academia. Aerospace companies familiar with developing aircraft and military instrumentation were often the developers, and they in turn subcontracted work to industry specialists, as warranted. Hybridization of commercial devices was done whenever feasible, with special packaging and testing for space flight often done by NASA. Intensive biomedical monitoring and research was done on the Skylab, the first space station, in 1973, but only relatively simple measurements could be made. Problems with attachment of surface sensors occurred throughout the mission, and needs for wireless biotelemetry data were apparent.

The innovation and invention processes of the early years continued in the 1980s and 1990s with increasing realization that the high costs and long development times for medical devices were becoming prohibitive. NASA increasingly wanted more involvement in defining the requirements and development process to optimize the reuse and upgrade capability of medical devices for the rapidly evolving Space Shuttle Program. Hybridized medical devices were increasingly used for human medical support and biomedical research. The first Spacelab, which allowed significant biomedical monitoring, flew in 1983 with several life sciences experiments. An industry-built miniaturized mass spectrometer for making gas metabolism measurements was developed and flown by NASA.

Today, as NASA continues to work on the International Space Station and plan for longer duration space travel, it is essential that the latest advances in technology are developed and applied to the new research objectives. Next-generation medical devices that will utilize emerging technologies—such as nanoscale devices, MEMS (micro-electromechanical systems), biosensors, gene arrays, biomimetics, robotics, advanced optics, and wireless communications—are under active study or are in development. Increasingly, collaboration by NASA with government, industry, and academic partners will be essential for co-development of dual-use medical devices. This process is driven by the need to take advantage of new clinical and biomedical measurements and to meet NASA's objectives in its Human Exploration and Development of Space program. NASA's programs for ATD and Technology Infusion will be essential for providing appropriate new medical devices on a schedule that will allow utilization in the era of the International Space Station.

ENDOVASCULAR DEVICES
Thomas J. Fogarty, M.D.
Professor of Surgery
Stanford University School of Medicine

Technology development as applied to surgical therapeutics, rather than just device technology alone, involves procedures, devices, instruments, techniques, drugs, and services. Transplantation provides a good example, as it certainly would not be possible without the availability of anti-rejection drugs.

One area of device development that relates to less invasive approaches is endovascular technology, which can be divided into diagnostics and therapeutics. In 1929, the concept of injecting dye into the vascular system was introduced by Dos Santos, who used the technique to outline tumors to understand their blood supply. Later, Forsman came up with a concept of coaxial catheter. It was introduced in the vascular system essentially to monitor some physiological parameters, and he actually used it on himself. Forsman was followed by Soames, who was interested in the pathology of a particular patient group with heart disease. By accident, he injected dye in the supervalvular position, and when the catheter was in the coronary he ended up doing a selective coronary catheterization. His peers thought it was an anecdotal occurrence without real impact on the field of medicine.

The next era involved catheter-mediated therapeutics to address acute arterial occlusions. The concept was developed by a scrub technician who worked on enough cases to know that when somebody had an acute arterial occlusion there are usually three operations. One was the attempt to get the occlusion out, which ultimately failed. The second was the amputation, usually below the knee, and then third was an amputation above the knee. This observation was based on no real critical science. The use and improvement of catheters was not perceived by the medical community or the device industry as significant events. The developers of these early devices were not well acknowledged by traditional medicine at the time, and their papers were not accepted by peer-reviewed journals.

What was viewed as insignificant has led to treatment of aneurysms with stent grafts, as well as treatment of trauma and congenital malformations such as A/V fistulas. I do not think anyone really conceived where this was going to go. As technology is applied to surgical therapeutics there rarely is a major paradigm shift; rather, change occurs slowly. Thus, medical technology as applied to surgical therapeutics involves many iterations in which the ultimate utility is inherently unpredictable. Technology is the application knowingly or unknowingly of documented science for practical purposes, for clinical utility. Certainly technology relies on science, and in some ways science does not move forward without certain technological innovations. Science is premised on theory, whereas technology is concerned with applications and utility. Technology may have implications for the company, the patient, or the physician who is employing it, but it is a very individual and personalized thing and science is rarely that.

How does one regulate innovation? A subject that currently presents significant confusion between regulatory agencies and drug and device manufacturers is the approach to safety and efficacy evaluation of these two very dissimilar products. There is a need to establish appropriate parameters for evaluating these entities. Recent interest in using an endovascular approach to manage carotid pathology has spurred great debate within the vascular surgical and radiological interventional community.

In relation to moving medical device innovation forward researchers must look at the processes currently being employed to evaluate devices as these methods can significantly impact the rate, quantity, and quality of device development.

A subject that currently presents significant confusion between regulatory agencies and drug and device manufacturers is the approach to safety and efficacy evaluations of these two very dissimilar products. There is a need to establish appropriate parameters for evaluating these entities.

Several years ago the FDA initiated sweeping changes to the regulatory process that effectively buried *device evaluations* under the identical regulations imposed for approval of *drug entities.* This attempt to apply a drug testing method to device testing is a seriously erroneous and inappropriate approach. In the development and assessment of drugs versus devices there are numerous distinct differences in these two therapeutic modalities, which highlight the inappropriateness of subjecting them to the same study methods. The influence of technique, significance of *in vitro* study, rate of technical change and the ability to visualize "real time" performance are all rated *low* for drugs while these parameters are considered *high* for devices. Conversely, the resources of the developer, cost development, and the duration of the regulatory cycle are *high* for drugs and generally *low* for devices. Device changes are iterative and rapid, unlike drug regimens, which can be titrated then set into concrete dosage forms. Devices, instrumentation, and specialized treatment systems must continually be refined and changed along the process route, which invariable does not lend itself to prospective randomized testing models.

In most cases, device evaluations utilizing prospective randomized clinical trials prove *not* to be the most advantageous method for determining efficacy because prospective randomization, in order to be valid, makes the following assumptions;

1. Case selection.
2. Technical competence and judgment is equal among all.
3. Diagnostic and monitoring modalities are frozen in time and are technician-insensitive, and interpretive skills are equal among all.
4. There is no prior fund of knowledge or reference points that are valid.
5. Post-procedure care is equivalent under all circumstances and the same in all institutions.
6. Intuition is of no importance in determining outcomes.
7. Improvements in technique, instruments, and implants have been optimized and are stabilized.
8. Assumes patient will cooperate in randomized treatment assignment scheme.
9. Enabling technology has stabilized.

To add to this list researchers must consider the medical ethical considerations inherent in randomizing patients into a treatment group. Patients who may best benefit from the new treatment modality may be eliminated from the trial protocol if they are not considered suitable candidates for the surgical alternative due to co-morbidities or psychological considerations.

Because valid historical controls exist, the technology is not stabilized, case selection is in a state of flux, and significant learning curves can influence results, attempts to use *only* randomized controlled studies to assess devices become inappropriate. Prospective randomization does not always answer the question when outcomes are unknown and clinical judgment is lacking. Clinical studies should be time- and cost-efficient, and credible. Prospective randomization represents only *one* method that can meet these criteria, and very often it is not the *best* method for obtaining an answer.

GENE ARRAYS
Stephen P.A. Fodor, Ph.D.
Chairman and Chief Executive Officer
Affymetrix

There are roughly three billion base pairs in the human genome. A huge multinational and multicorporate effort to sequence the genome will produce a first rough draft in 2001. But the sequence alone is not enough. Researchers need to know not just the base-pair sequence, but also the function of those sequences and how variation affects function. Which genes are turned on and off under different circumstances? What are the polymorphisms? What are the differences from individual to individual?

The technology developed at Affymetrix is the so-called "DNA chip." The chip uses some of the tricks of the semiconductor industry, photolithography, and combinatorial chemical synthesis and some detection technologies. A lithographic mask shines light in certain areas of the chip, activating the surface, which is flooded with reagents to build DNA molecules. These chips are not made one at a time, but in wafers, like semiconductors. A chip about the size of a dime can hold up to 400,000 different pieces of DNA at precise locations on the surface.

The basic idea of the chip is that one adds a patient sample with a fluorescent tag. As it incubates with a single strand of DNA it will find its complementary structure on the chip and bond. The fluorescent tag allows the DNA to be read using a confocal scanning system made by Hewlett-Packard. The chips are disposable, and there is software that goes with the system. Much of the early development of the technology was funded by small companies and federal research agencies.

The technology allows for numerous comparisons. For example, a sequence that matches up with normal wild-type DNA shows one sort of pattern of fluorescence, and if a mutation is present the pattern changes, which can be detected very easily. This allows for the detection of disease-causing or predisposing mutations, such as P53, BRCA-1, and BRCA-2. There is a chip to look at some of the genes in HIV to monitor drug resistance, and others to find the presence of a strain of virus or bacteria, based on a piece of its DNA. Nearly 400,000 probes can be placed on a chip, which allows information to be processed simultaneously, an important tool for the human genome project. This is especially useful for the study of polymorphisms, or genetic differences between people. It turns out that there is about one in every 1,000 base pairs that varies across individuals. These single nucleotide polymorphisms, or SNPs, usually have no clinical implications, but serve as a means to identify similarities and differences among people and populations. Chips and powerful statistical genetics provide the opportunity to pursue SNPs as markers for disease as well as for the application of pharmacogenetics.

In 1995, Affymetrix took the entire human mitochondrial genome, 16,500 base pairs, and put it on a chip. The subsequent large-scale polymorphism scanning project with Eric Lander at the Whitehead Institute found 3,000 SNPs throughout the genome, which were mapped to different chromosomes. This capability will lead to better prediction and diagnosis of disease, but also the ability to trace population migrations and family history. Subtle variations might also explain human preferences, for example, preference or aversion to specific smells. It also allows one to look at banks of genes, for example, related to hypertension or cancer, and understand which genes turn off or on in disease. One can develop drugs that target that action.

INHALED INSULIN
Robert B. Chess
Chief Executive Officer
Inhale Therapeutic Systems, Inc.

Many of the drugs being developed through biotechnology—insulin, erythropoietin, growth hormone, and interferon—are essentially protein products, and the common problem with these drugs is that the only way to administer them is by injection. If one takes them as pills they are broken down by the gastrointestinal system. They are too large to enter through the stomach or through the nose or skin. One alternative is to administer them through the lung, and if one gets them down to the deep lung, to the alveoli, most of them flow into the bloodstream. This is the technological premise of advanced inhalables technology from Inhale Therapeutic Systems, Inc. (San Carlos, Calif).

Inhale Therapeutic Systems, Inc. is a drug delivery development company with a platform of technologies. The researchers there do not develop the drug products themselves but partner with biotechnology and large pharmaceutical companies. These partners typically lead the clinical development and market the product; Inhale Therapeutic Systems, Inc. provides the technology to allow them to do this and then manufacture it once the product is developed. Inhale has 400 employees, including mechanical and chemical engineers, aerosol scientists, physicists, and protein chemists. In 10 years, Inhale has initiated 12 different financings.

Inhale's lead inhalable product is developing a better system for insulin delivery. Inhalable insulin is less invasive than injections and might increase compliance and adherence to treatment. A large NIH-sponsored trial followed 1,400 people over 9 years: some took insulin twice a day and others took it three to six times a day. The study found that those who took insulin three to six times a day decreased the side effects of diabetes by 35 to 60%. Side effects include blindness, the need for lower body amputations, and coronary failure. One out of seven health care dollars—$100 billion a year—is spent on diabetes care. Despite that study, only 15 percent of patients have adopted the increased dosage, most likely because the injections are painful. Inhalable insulin offers an easy alternative.

The reason that inhalable insulin has not been developed to date is the difficulty of getting drugs to reach the deep lung so that they can be absorbed efficiently into the bloodstream. Inhale has pioneered the pulmonary delivery technology to enable the delivery of these delicate macromolecules through the lung. The first step was to make the particles stable at 1 to 5 microns in size. The challenge was to formulate the powders so that they are as chemically and physically stable as the day they were made and can deliver the same product six months later. Researchers used glass stabilization to pack the particles so they are not moving around and so that the protein is not coming in contact with the water of the particles. The final product is very stable in a wide range of temperatures, which is a great convenience for those with diabetes as they will not have to refrigerate the drug.

To process the powdered drugs, researchers had to modify conventional spray drying used in food processing to make the small particles. It is the first time that any company has used spray drying on this scale to make particles this fine and in the process researchers had to keep the consistency of the particles the same for each level of scaling up to the next output size.

Another challenge was filling the particles in individual dose units. Researchers needed different dose strengths, because individuals must titrate their dose.

To help drive the drug into the deep lung where it needs to be delivered to enable systemic delivery, researchers developed a unique delivery inhaler. Because drug particles need to be delivered consistently from person to person, researchers could not rely on patients' inspiratory flow rate so they developed an inhaler that operates independently of a patient's inhaling flow rate. Clinical trials have indicated that reproducibility is as good as, if not better than, the injection approach.

Phase II and Phase III clinical trials have been encouraging and patients have expressed satisfaction with this new delivery method that is breaking new ground.

IMAGING THE MICROVASCULATURE
Richard Nadeau, Ph.D.
Chairman and Chief Executive Officer
Cytometrics, Inc.

Cytometrics was founded in 1992. The mission of Cytometrics is to commercialize noninvasive, point-of-care products, using the Company's patented *OPS Imaging* technology for direct observation and measurement of the microcirculatory system and surrounding tissue. For example, by inserting a probe under the tongue, individual blood cells can be visualized. This allows one to do a complete blood count, hemoglobin, and hematocrit, noninvasively. In newborns the device can be used directly on the skin. When it is applied to the conjunctiva of an adult diabetic, the distinct irregularities in the microvascular structure are clear. Also, the device can be used during surgery to observe the microvasculature of various organs, such as the liver, heart, and lung. The microvascular structure is very characteristic and different for different organs. Irregularities are powerful predictors of disease.

The Cytoscan Video Microscope is an OPS imaging platform: it has an optical probe, a computer, a light source, and software to operate the instrument. The device takes two high-quality polarizers and crosses them. A small percentage of the polarized light undergoes multiple scattering events as it penetrates into the material or the subject, and during that process the light becomes depolarized. The only reflected light observed is the depolarized light, which effectively is created inside the material, and which has back illuminated the blood vessels. In effect, this optical design creates a virtual light source inside the subject, even though the light is in front of the subject.

The Cytoscan is designed primarily for visualization of the microcirculation. It is Class I FDA exempt, and will be marketed in Europe and the United States. Model II, available in 2001, will have more extensive image analysis capabilities. A desirable computation capability being developed is to measure a functional capillary index, or the amount of blood flowing within a tissue along with its hemoglobin concentration.

Clinical observations of the microvascular structure have been made by inserting the optical probe into the rectum for the differential diagnosis of Crohn's disease and ulcerative colitis. Also, the device has been tested comparing normal subjects sublingually with subjects in cardiogenic or septic shock. In cardiogenic shock, the large vessels are almost empty, and more importantly, in the small vessels there is virtually no flow. Capillary flow is either sluggish or completely stopped; this also occurs following cardiac bypass and in some cases of stroke. In septic shock, there is hypervelocity flow in the larger vessels, and again slow flow or no flow in the small vessels.

Further, the Cytoscan has been used in the context of neurosurgery, in individuals being operated on for cerebral hemorrhages. In 4 out of the 12, or 14 cases to date, microvascular spasms were observed; these patients later died, suggesting that the spasms require early aggressive treatment.

The company founders put $1.6 million of their own money into the company to get the device through the very early seed phase. That allowed them to do proof of concept *in vitro*. They then attempted to raise money through contracts, venture capital, and technology incubators, all of which proved to be ineffective. The company was forced to raise its own funds, privately.

In the seed phase, raising funds was the greatest obstacle for Cytometrics. The federal and state grants and contract systems were too slow, too bureaucratic, and too much trouble for too little money. Moreover, incubators want to own the intellectual property. A solution would be to improve the government role in seed funding. In order to receive federal funding, universities should be required to establish technology incubators and provide an environment in which technologies can be nurtured, particularly in the early critical phases. Added tax incentives for investment would help raise capital for early-stage, high-risk companies.

The development stage poses a different set of problems that are more regulatory and legal. These obstacles are higher in the United States; thus, many companies do their initial testing in Europe. In effect, most U.S. companies are exporting their technology. Some remedy could come if U.S. legislation were enacted limiting liability for clinical trials, and if there were more industry involvement in the design and implementation of government regulations.

GENERAL DISCUSSION OF THE NATURE OF MEDICAL INNOVATION

Discussion of this session's talks began with a question about whether the Cytoscan imaging system had been used in the capillary bed in the nose, where one could gain access to two of the four major arteries that serve the brain.

Richard Nadeau answered that the current probe is a little shorter and thicker than he would like, but it is only the first generation. Cytometrics would very much like a longer, thinner probe that could be used in the nose or be curved around the back of the heart. If they had $100 million they would definitely develop a second-generation probe like that, but the priority at the moment is to get the basic product launched.

Clifford Goodman, chairing the session, then asked Robert Chess to expand on one of the lessons learned that he had mentioned, namely, whether he actually had to stop the innovative process so that he would not upset the regulatory review. Mr. Chess responded that that was correct. He had to continue improvements in parallel, while freezing the initial insulin product to keep the regulatory approval process rolling. For example, he said, they learned in late 1997 that if they made their particles a slightly different way they could improve the efficiency of the system by a factor of two, which would be very important both for the cost of goods for the product and the cost of the product for the patients. It probably would not have made any difference clinically, but they would have needed to repeat probably a year's worth of trials, so they decided not to do it. They are now hoping to convince their partner, Pfizer, to start some clinical trials with the improved version in about a year or a year and a half, and then introduce a more efficient version a year or two later. The net effect is to slow the stream of innovation and leave patient care lagging significantly behind the capabilities the technology could provide. Mr. Chess also pointed out that the decision to pursue improvements on a parallel track was one a less well-financed company would not have been able to make, delaying innovation still further.

Thomas Fogarty from Stanford pointed out that some of the recent changes in FDA have allowed innovations based upon experience in Phase I and Phase II without going back. For example, he said, when some mechanical parameters were obviously marginal very early in Phase I, FDA permitted the necessary changes without mandate that the study be restarted. That was something he would not have expected 5 to 7 years ago.

Dean Kamen provided a second example of how regulation can slow the pace of innovation, drawing on his development of a robotic wheelchair substitute and noting that he is amazed at how well the regulatory people "get it" when one talks to them individually, but how the process and the rules that they have to follow cause trouble nonetheless. Mr. Kamen recounted that 9 years ago when he started building his robot, he did not care what the gyros cost for his proof of concept, so he bought aerospace gyros at $2,000 apiece. They are big and delicate, but he crammed them in, and only used two, since he did not need redundancy just to check the system. For a production machine he planned to get super reliability through redundant architecture, and put in six gyros, monitoring all of them with redundant processes. He also knew that the price would be brought down by using some solid-state gyros that cost a few hundred dollars, so he started trials. He monitored the auto industry, however, and soon discovered that two major suppliers to the automotive industry built a whole subassembly of solid-state gyros for use in advanced systems like the detonation devices on air bags. Because they are making them by the millions it turns out they are $10 apiece and incredibly robust. It also does not matter if something goes wrong with them because of the redundancy in Kamen's design—with six gyros, one failure would not negatively impact the machine. When he tried to put these new gyros in, though, he discovered that, since the gyro is listed as a critical component of the device, he would have to redo all their system level testing. That would take a year, cost a few million dollars. As a result, he is about to launch the product with a set of gyros that will add $200 to the final selling price of the machine, knowing for the last 2 years that he must wait for the next generation of product to incorporate an individual component that might legally fit the description of critical, but is not critical at all because of the system architecture. He concluded that the approval system has to evolve to where good engineering judgment is what dictates what makes the product safe rather than a process that was designed at a different time.

Kshitij Mohan started the discussion on a second major thread by asking about the value of the degree of exclusivity, the protection of patent-like quality, that FDA approval grants to a technology.

Dr. Nadeau replied that he hated to use the regulatory process as a barrier to entry, since everyone here is in the business of helping patients, and if one does that one is not helping patients, because that tends to exclude smaller companies.

Steven Fodor proffered that the dilemma is not limited to just the FDA process. Once someone is shown how to do something it is always easier for that person to do it again, and big companies particularly often will not pay for the start-up risk of many of the technologies discussed today. Once other people are shown how to do it, they tend to compete with you, and that brings up the nature of our whole patent system and being able to protect one's innovations.

Dr. Nadeau talked about the pros and cons of the Patent Cooperation Treaty (PCT) in response to a question about the getting a "world patent." He reported that his company generally filed PCT applications first, because the PCT examiners who do the search are professional searchers, whereas in the United States the examiner does both the search and the examination. As a result, the PCT applicant gets a preliminary report and a really good idea of what the patent literature is, which is a terrific advantage for a later filing in the United States.

Dean Kamen added that "world patent" is unfortunately somewhat of a misnomer, since U.S. inventors can get patents in India, China, and even places as close as Brazil and Mexico, which happily take your money, but will not enforce the patents, or even let the patent holders enforce them very effectively. As a practical matter though, he said, the PCT has been a big improvement. One can file here in the PCT and, at least for the first year, buy the protection for the initial period of testing and evaluation. It is expensive though, and his company has spent a lot more than $500,000 protecting its core technologies.

Another member of the group added that one of the problems a small company faces is raising money to do the development, and a key to that is having clinicians present at medical meetings to describe their experiences with the product. That puts it out in the public arena, however, and hurts chances for a patent. A company can get a basic patent on the PCT or in the United States, but the development process here and the issues of doing the iterative changes all take time. All it takes is a doctor in Europe to say, "Hey, that is a brilliant idea; go get an engineer," and they will end up getting blocking patents. So, despite spending a fortune, foreign competitors will have a major role when the inventor wants to make that next change in his or her product. The intellectual property issue is a big issue when you tie it to the regulatory issue.

Dr. Goodman steered the discussion back to the FDA by asking Steve Fodor whether FDA regulations ever change a decision to pursue innovation, or whether the hurdle of Medicare coverage ever changes a decision about pursuing an innovation or how fast to do so. Dr. Fodor responded that when he first started this pursuing the DNA chip technology he had a lot of thoughts about genetic diagnostics, chips for cystic fibrosis or other diseases, but it turned out that precisely because of the FDA barriers, plus the difficulty of making a profit on those relatively small-market products, he had to make the decision to point the technology toward things that people could just not possibly do otherwise, that is, whole genome scanning, very broad-scale applications. The products that his company now makes are not under any sort of FDA regulatory approval process, except for things such as the HIV product and the p53 and cytochrome P450 chips. These three are focused on specific areas, but for those products he partners with companies like Roche Molecular Systems that have experience with the FDA.

Jean Harmon, from NIH, then asked about how to improve the Small Business Innovative Research (SBIR) program at the NIH, to which Dr Nadeau responded that the problem is that if one does the straight-line extension of the obvious one can get funding, but if one proposes anything that is innovative, that is unproven, then one cannot. He suggested that one way of solving that problem is similar to the way companies manage R&D budgets. They take a small percentage of their budget and they put it into high-risk areas, some additional percentage into less risky areas, and then finally another percentage into sure bets.

Mr. Kamen acknowledged that he had never received an SBIR grant, but recounted his amazement that so many small companies come to his firm with them, particularly people who have left universities. He has had four or five people come to his company over the years who literally have lived on SBIR grants for the last 10 years. They understand the process. They know how to get that money, he said, but the only other thing that is consistent about them is that the Darwinian system of the marketplace would have chewed them up. Kamen's suggestion for improvement: make the grant bigger and tell people, "You get one and only one. If you do what you said, great, you shouldn't need us anymore. If you didn't do what you said, shame on you."

Dr. Fodor took a contrary view, noting that his company had actually found the SBIR programs extremely effective, along with traditional R01 awards and National Institute of Standards and Technology (NIST) grants in the first few years of the company's existence.

Mr. Chess on the other hand, said his company looked into SBIR but decided not to bother, because they figured that if the work was important they should do it, and if it can wait 6 months for them to fill out the application and wait to hear back then it probably is not that important. And, at that time at least, the amount of money was so small it was not worth all the trouble. Dr. Nadeau closed the discussion by repeating the suggestion from his presentation about the idea of matching funds as is done in Germany. If the applicant puts up a dollar, he or she can get two. Maybe, he suggested, NIH should omit the elaborate applications and simply say, "If you have money, we will match it, two for one, and that is it."

4

Sources and Support of Medical Devices Innovation

Presenters in this session described and analyzed the sources and amount of resources available in the medical device innovation field; discussed the role of small, large, and multinational medical companies in medical device innovation; identified the issues and opportunities confronted by innovators in this field; described the role of standards and product applications; discussed the effects of venture capital on this field; and evaluated the role of the legal system in influencing innovation.

AN OVERVIEW OF PUBLIC AND PRIVATE FACTORS AFFECTING MEDICAL DEVICE INNOVATION
Clifford Goodman, Ph.D.
Senior Scientist
The Lewin Group

Sources and timing of support for medical device innovation can be viewed in the context of the medical device life cycle, which can be described in five main streams or pathways of activity: (1) regulation, (2) research and development, (3) manufacturing, (4) marketing, and (5) legal. Medical device innovators and manufacturers increasingly look downstream to the sequence and height of the hurdles along these interrelated pathways to inform their decisions to continue development of a device, modify it, divert resources to other products, or otherwise alter the process of innovation. Continued pursuit of innovation when these hurdles are not aligned or harmonized can require considerable corporate resources, adding risk to the prospects for innovation. Venture capitalists and other investors consider where an emerging technology is in these streams of activity, and what its prospects are for overcoming these hurdles, when deciding whether to invest in the technology.

The regulatory pathway is generally well defined, with certain parallels between the United States and Europe. Some of the main benchmarks in the United States are design controls; investigational device exemptions (IDE) for devices requiring clinical (human) testing, which requires institutional review board (IRB) approval; premarketing approval (PMA); good manufacturing practices (GMPs); and various forms of medical device reporting once a device is on the market. There are analogs to these hurdles in Europe, for example, the CE mark, which is the market clearance hurdle in much the same manner as the PMA in the United States. Still, the requirements for a CE mark and a U.S. PMA, and the accompanying paperwork, are likely to differ, necessitating resource expenditures for companies seeking international markets for their products.

Although the R&D pathway is anchored by iterative design, preclinical testing, and development of device prototypes, there are other important benchmarks along the way. These include permission to conduct clinical testing (granted by, e.g., the IDE in the regulatory pathway); clinical evaluation (leading to market approval in the marketing pathway); outcomes and health economic research to persuade payers, technology assessment agencies, and others of the worthiness of the technology; and postmarket research and surveillance to gather data about the experience of the device in the field, which helps to fulfill regulatory requirements and provides information for further marketing efforts. One of the challenges in the medical technology industry in the more developed nations is that most new technologies do not result in obvious gains in mortality or morbidity, so that it is important to demonstrate improvements in quality of life and economic advantages. Further, more health care providers and payers want to see evidence of effectiveness in community settings rather than just efficacy in the carefully controlled settings that characterize data gathering for purposes of regulatory approval.

The marketing pathway often starts with market research on user needs, competition, and other factors that can influence device design as well as the regulatory and R&D pathways to be taken by the technology, including what types of health and economic evidence will be required to demonstrate the value of the technology. Education and promotion of the device can begin even before market approval, preparing the target markets and informing those who will be in a position to order and use the device. Sales, distribution, and customer support functions must be in place upon market approval. Third-party payment, which usually depends on market approval by regulators and can be further influenced by other evidence from outcomes research and health economics studies, can strongly mediate sales. Helping device users with third-party payment can be critical. Some companies have established 800 numbers for physicians to call if they are having problems with procedure coding or other aspects of reimbursement for use of the device.

In parallel to the other streams of activity, companies must gear up their manufacturing capacity. This includes facility requirements, maintaining the flow of materials and components, the production process, quality management, and ongoing modifications and retooling of the manufacturing process as needed to cope with device redesign, swings in demand for the device, and other changes.

Legal considerations must be managed throughout the device life cycle, including gaining patents, licensing, maintaining patient protection, and protecting against product liability.

In contrast to the pharmaceutical industry, the medical device industry is characterized by a large number of small entrepreneurial companies and start-ups. While these companies are largely focused on gaining "proof of concept" and overcoming initial regulatory hurdles, they tend not to have the staff size, experience, and other resources needed to manage these different pathways in the device life cycle. Further, since they tend not to have broad product lines that can sustain their cash flow, their risk profile is more closely tied to the success of one or a few products. As such, the viability of these companies is highly sensitive to changes in regulatory hurdles, payment requirements, sales and distribution, manufacturing capacity, legal challenges, and other factors that can divert their limited resources. These factors tend to influence the points at which small companies are more amenable to being acquired by larger ones or to engaging in other partnerships that will provide the resources needed to manage these requirements.

Current patterns of public- and private-sector funding for R&D, particularly for basic research in the sciences and engineering underlying medical device development, affect the nature and flow of new technology. Aside from traditional funding sources for R&D, changes in payment criteria are providing some earlier revenue streams that can improve the risk outlook for innovation. These are exemplified by various "conditional coverage" arrangements for investigational technology, such as the 1995 Health Care Financing Administration/FDA interagency agreement on reimbursement of investigational medical devices, and greater collaboration of research agencies and health care payers to support clinical trials and other studies of investigational technologies.

THE FEDERAL RESEARCH ROLE
John T. Watson, Ph.D.
Acting Deputy Director
National Heart, Lung and Blood Institute

The NIH Revitalization Act of 1993 included language (the so-called Durenburger Amendment) requiring the DHHS Secretary to report on "Support for Bioengineering Research." The study included an inventory of federal bioengineering support, a non-federal consultant working group, an evaluation of patenting trends for implantable prostheses, an estimate of non-profit and for-profit support for bioengineering research, and an open workshop to access all findings and make recommendations to NIH. The term "bioengineering" was used in its broadest context, in terms of medicine and biology.

This report led to congressional inquiries about its conclusions. In response, NIH, under the leadership of Director Harold Varmus, formed the NIH Bioengineering Consortium (BECON) in 1997. Simultaneously, many groups increasingly recognized the need for bioengineering support, including the Whitaker Foundation, the American Institute for Medical and Biological Engineering, the Small Business Innovation Research Program, and the NIST Advanced Technology Program. The interests of groups collectively demonstrated the growing importance and awareness of the central role of bioengineering to innovation and invention in medical and biological research and clinical procedures.

The NIH and the Consultant Report recommended some sort of central NIH focus for bioengineering. Support for basic bioengineering research, contrasted to applied and developmental research, was reported as 30% of the total, compared to an NIH average of 60% for all other fields. These reports also addressed the need for an evaluation of the NIH peer-review process for bioengineering research, membership on advisory committees, the movement of new device introduction overseas, the biomaterials availability problem, uncertainties in the innovation process, and using patent information to trace back to related federal research support. Finally, regulation must be meshed with innovation so that entrepreneurs can figure out a way to meet the regulatory guidance in a more cost-effective and shorter time frame.[1]

THE FEDERAL REGULATORY ROLE
Susan Alpert, M.D., Ph.D.
Director, Center for Food Safety and Applied Nutrition
Food and Drug Administration

Regulatory oversight of medical products is an accepted part of the government's role in providing protection of the public health. At the same time, governmental acceptance of a technology or product contributes to broader acceptance and reliance on the claims of the product's provider. The threshold that innovations cross to reach the market sets in place an important foundation. This foundation must be established on the basis of good scientific principles and data to have its intended impact—benefit to the public health without undue delay.

The actual interface of the regulatory agencies in the federal government and the innovators in medical device technology and products is broad. There are far-reaching areas of impact, such as those resulting from the development and recognition of technical consensus standards that may be used in design, manufacturing, or regulatory activities. There are specific and more limited areas of impact, such as the individual developer's meetings with the scientific and regulatory staff of an agency, which focus on details of the information to

---

[1] Subsequent to the workshop, NIH established the National Institute of Biomedical Imaging and Bioengineering (NIBIB).

be submitted and evaluated for market entry or reimbursement, for example. The impact on device innovation from activities at each of these levels and those in between must be acknowledged and evaluated.

Given the focus on government spending by regulatory agencies for programs seen to be beyond their specific mandate, and which might present conflict of interest, the type of financial support that can be provided to the industry is limited in this sector. There are programs, however, that may be used to broadly enhance the development of new technologies while being responsive to concerns regarding a level playing field among competing companies. In addition, the tasks of the regulatory agencies should, and frequently do, include (1) providing pathways to market that are responsive to the changing timeframes for technology and product development, (2) creating processes that are sufficiently flexible to facilitate novel product development, and (3) incentives for innovators whose product provides a significant contribution to the public health.

There are tensions in place between the need for and the speed of introduction of the new technologies and products. There is a need for better communication between the large companies and the small innovators. Regulation is a necessary obstacle because society demands some type of oversight and accountability. FDA is charged by the public to ensure that device market entry involves products that are both safe and effective. FDA publishes summaries of safety and effectiveness data for devices so that it can be made clear and transparent as to what this product is, and what can be expected from it.

THE ACADEMIC ROLE IN INNOVATION
John A. Parrish, M.D.
Center for Integration of Medicine and Innovative Technology
Massachusetts General Hospital

Academia has much to offer the field of medical device innovation, including "problem-rich" and "solution-rich" environments, "molecular" understanding of pathophysiology and mechanisms of therapy, expertise and skills, access to patients, and a culture of scientific methodology.

There are multiple barriers intrinsic to most academic institutions that limit the development of diagnostic and therapeutic devices. There is often a large cultural and psychological gap between the disciplines of biology and engineering that prevents effective dialogue. This results in a lack of clear understanding of clinical problems by the technologist, lack of awareness about technical options by clinicians, and difficulty finding appropriate collaborations. Within the academic medical community, specialization has been a powerful force in learning more about individual diseases and organ systems but has also resulted in turf wars in patient care, destructive competition, and poor communication.

One model for enhancing the role of academia is the Center for Integration of Medicine and Innovative Technology (CIMIT), a collaboration of academic physicians and engineers working with industry and government to solve important medical problems. The founding institutions can be considered as the problem-rich environments (the teaching hospitals of Harvard Medical School) and the solution-rich environments (Massachusetts Institute of Technology and Charles Draper Labs). The mission is to improve patient care by bringing together technologists, engineers, scientists, and clinicians to catalyze development of innovative technology, emphasizing minimally invasive diagnoses and therapy. CIMIT is led by senior academicians whose full-time commitment is to integrate technology into health care by systematic, non-random purposeful mixing and matching of appropriate clinical champions and engineering experts. The process is intended to:

- identify difficult health care problems amenable to technological solutions,
- encourage teams of clinicians and engineers to generate new solutions,
- provide resources to develop solutions for safer and more efficacious treatments, and
- facilitate the application, transfer and commercialization of CIMIT technology.

CIMIT provides funds to develop and demonstrate new ideas and expertise to guide the development of commercializable products. This expertise includes:

- business development,
- technology development,
- regulation affairs, reimbursement issues,
- patient safety, simulation, and
- industry liaison programs.

Longitudinal programs include development of selected technologies (e.g., devices, tissue engineering, imaging) and focus on selected clinical problems ripe for new technological solutions (e.g., acute stroke management, identification and treatment of vulnerable plaque).

Success is measured by scientific presentations, published papers, patents, and receipt of NIH grants. There is also evidence that CIMIT support for numerous multidisciplinary projects and programs resulted in outcomes that would not have occurred absent that support. Dedicated funding is essential: there is no better way to get people's attention.

THE ACADEMIC HEALTH CENTER ENVIRONMENT
Robert W. Anderson, M.D.
David C. Sabiston Professor and Chair
Department of Surgery
Duke University

Health care incentives have been perverse for many years. There are high prices with overcapacity, common technology is extremely expensive, and we support mediocrity in clinical care and technology development. Researchers have encouraged the use of health care services because of the fee-for-service mentality, and researchers have failed to promote health and wellness.

There is a tremendous competitiveness in the market. Purchasers have been more sophisticated with an emphasis on cost, often at the expense of technology and innovation. Unlike other industries that blossomed in recent years with high initial start-up costs with a lot of capitalization—and shrinking prices as volume grew—prices only recently shrank in health care.

Shifting sites of care toward more outpatient services has increased. This change has produced technology expenses due to improper use and overuse. Moreover, pharmaceutical spending is on the rise. The factors that are driving change are economics, outcomes and evidence-based medicine, new technology, preventive medicine, and new procedures. Evidence-based and outcomes-based medicine are going to lead to greater accountability and possibly risk-based reimbursement.

New technologies, for example, molecular biology, gene therapy, organ substitution, stem cell biology, and smart devices, will allow researchers to identify high-risk groups of patients and, in many instances, start treatment to prevent onset of disease. New minimally invasive procedures have tremendous potential.

Other factors that researchers need to consider in innovation and health are changing demographics, in particular the aging of the United States population. The number of elderly and disabled Medicare beneficiaries is growing rapidly. In addition, the growth of the uninsured—48.7 million people in the year 2000 in the United States—poses real challenges to the health of the nation.

What can the device industry learn from other industries? First, short-term solutions do not sustain survival. Second, competition creates value. Third, innovation drives continuous quality improvement, and fourth, incentives drive innovation. The problem with determining quality is that no one has adequately defined its parameters. The basic elements for health care change are going to be corrected incentives to improve efficiency, access to relevant information, and sophisticated information systems. As always, any player in the health care market had better be able to demonstrate improved clinical outcomes and cost-effectiveness.

Increasingly, teaching hospitals are the place where complex illness and procedures come together. Teaching hospitals provide care for more severely ill patients. More than half of all major teaching hospitals now have operating margins of less than 0%. As a result, there is a lot of cost cutting going on. The key success factors for academic health centers will be human and fiscal resources. Researchers have to continue to build on their human resources, getting the best people, and training and retaining them. Researchers have to shore up their fiscal resources.

Despite this, academic health centers retain great advantages for clinical trials. Researchers have access to patient populations, and have highly trained personnel. The disadvantages are cultural conflicts, limited capital, and, often, underdeveloped infrastructure. The hindrances to new product development have always been shortage of important new product ideas in certain areas. In addition, the new product development process is very expensive. Academic institutions must become better at working with industry while maintaining their freedom, and seeking non-traditional revenue sources.

THE ROLE OF SMALL MEDICAL COMPANIES
Thomas M. Loarie
Chief Executive Officer
Kera Vision, Inc.

The product Loarie has been involved with for the last 13 years is a device for correcting common vision problems. It is two half rings made of biocompatible polymer that can be inserted into the periphery of the cornea. It stays outside the optical zone and reshapes the cornea so one can get the light rays to fall on the retina. The product can be removed, and in most cases the eye goes back to its original status. This device received FDA approval in 1999. Researchers raised $160 million to bring this to market, making this probably the largest up-front investment in history for medical technology. It is ultimately the public that will be the judge of whether or not researchers are doing their job.

The medical device industry includes 6,000 companies and 3,000 product lines covering 50 clinical specialties. There are only 64 product groups that have revenues over $150 million, and there are only 100 companies that have revenues over $100 million. Seventy-two percent of the medical device firms employ fewer than 50 people. This is really a cottage industry. In global terms, there is great competition. A sustainable advantage by any company can only be attained by leveraging knowledge.

The aging of the population will place demands on this health care system. Technology becomes an important player in helping to solve a dilemma that is before researchers in the very near future. It is the small companies that drive innovation, yet out of 60 ideas, only one product actually makes it to the marketplace, so this is a very fragile process, one that is challenged by the typical mentality of investors. In most areas of the United States, in venture capital there are only two things that are important, feasibility and market acceptance. The regulatory and health care payment environments introduce additional levels of uncertainty. Small companies are agile, with a tremendous tolerance for ambiguity, and are therefore well suited to be the source of innovation for medical devices.

THE ROLE OF LARGE MEDICAL COMPANIES
John P. Wareham
Chief Executive Officer
Beckman Coulter, Inc.

Beckman Coulter, Inc. makes products that patients do not see and physicians seldom see—that is, genetic analysis systems, drug discovery enabling systems, and diagnostic systems used by laboratorians. One of the things that researchers do is make available technologies that can be used to create value in the marketplace. Every medical device company, whether large or small, is focused on bringing real-life patient utility to technology. The unique contribution of a large company is that it can address the development imperative.

Once a technology is invented, bringing it to the point where it can be commercialized requires capital, along with certain competencies and management processes. Large companies are involved in discovery and commercialization processes. The special role of large companies is to contribute infrastructure, market knowledge, and financial resources to validate technologies and make them valuable to patients.

This is a very complex time in history, and a large medical company has the internal resources to help deal with this complexity. For example, in the not too distant future researchers might expect to run a diagnostic test that identifies a gene protein or cell profile that enables a physician to prescribe a course of treatment. While this is the direction of the genomic revolution, policy and regulatory requirements will add layers of complexity to such a capability. These issues, combined with concerns about health care cost management, may drive some innovation into the realm of large companies. Cost management concerns are driving more automation, product standardization, systems integration, and information management, all of which can eventually drive costs up.

It is vitally important for large companies to capture and quantify patient outcomes so that researchers can fairly assess the economic impact of health care technologies. If researchers are lowering costs by preventing disease and more effective monitoring and treatment of disease, then investments in innovation are being made well.

All of these innovations have the potential to control health care costs and improve quality, but there is another factor at play, consumerism. Patients, as consumers of health care, are becoming more informed. They are demanding better information, choices of treatment options, and control. Individuals want to know why tests are ordered, what the results mean, and how they can monitor their own health and prevent disease. As individuals become more involved in their own health care, there will be even a greater demand for information and technology. This drives up costs.

Large medical device companies have the ability to bring scale to the challenge of globalization and successful product development. In a global business environment, the small incubators of technology are particularly challenged with respect to financial pressures. While small companies lack the infrastructure to take on worldwide development and marketing activity, large companies have the infrastructure to help small companies get their technology to patients around the globe. Large companies can supply capital and credibility. In fact, large companies are already playing a key role in the growth of the medical device industry through acquisition, joint ventures, strategic alliances, contract research, licensing, and royalty agreements.

Mergers and acquisitions in supplies, equipment, and devices grew dramatically over the last five years, from $5 billion in 1994 to $32 billion in 1998. Despite this, large companies will continue to rely on smaller startups for their ideas and inventions. At Beckman Coulter, this has led to externalizing technology innovation. The objective was to spend half of the budget for technology innovation in collaborative agreements. This may involve a number of parties, including small companies, institutes, academia, and contract research organizations. In this model, researchers use their capital and credibility to build teams that are necessary to assess and pursue these worthy causes, with a net result of bringing utility to patients faster. To sum up, large medical companies have the capital, competency, and management processes to fulfill the development imperative.

THE ROLE OF PUBLIC AND PRIVATE CAPITAL
J. Casey McGlynn
Partner, Wilson, Sonsini, Goodrich and Rosati

The financial players in health care innovation have changed in recent years. The venture capital community, in particular, has changed over the past 20 years from diversified funds to organizations in which individuals have become more focused on particular technologies. In addition, a number of traditional investors in the health care field have left or disbanded their health care divisions. They turned away from health care because development time in the Internet area is so short and the returns are so staggering. In addition, the lack of returns from the biotechnology industry was discouraging. The percentage of venture capital dollars going into health care approximated a third to a half several years ago. Today it is about 10 to 12%. The medical device sector includes about 208 companies in the United States. In 1999 there were roughly 30 first rounds. These numbers are very small with little room for expansion.

Thus, diversified funds are not as sure a source of capital for entrepreneurs as they were in the past. Fortunately, corporations are more active in the venture world today than they were five years ago. They have become basic supporters of venture capital and one of the major stalwarts of getting companies funded and technology into the marketplace.

Incubators continue to be critically important. They are incredibly valuable to the doctor who might be the ultimate innovator but who lacks the needed resources to build infrastructure and get an idea transformed into reality. The number of incubators is on the rise, a positive development in the medical device industry.

Factors that challenge the device industry in terms of raising capital are long development time, regulation, and uncertainty about reimbursement. In addition, limited liquidity from the public sector limits venture capital's ability to guess predictably when it will turn a profit on an investment in the medical device industry. One area where initial public offerings have been on the rise in recent years is in genomics, in large part leveraged by the enormous investment made by the federal government in basic research in this field. Nevertheless, there are more venture capitalists interested in the medical device field than in the biotechnology field, probably because the science is not as complex and therefore the risks are clearer.

The emergence of E-health companies, for example, medical records, has drawn a lot of interest and capital but there are many companies all pursuing the same products. Big companies that are innovative are adopting Internet tools to make themselves more efficient. The small companies will be adopting those same kinds of products to speed up the collection of data, to make that data more precise, and to make regulatory filings quicker and easier.

GENERAL DISCUSSION OF SOURCES AND SUPPORT OF MEDICAL DEVICE INNOVATION

Tom Fogarty from Stanford began the discussion with a question contained in a story about a clinical trial involving carotid pathology. He was approached about participating in this multisite trial, he said, which upon close inspection turned out to be a brilliant effort to do something real stupid. When Dr. Fogarty called the individual responsible to ask why he was doing this and tell him why the trial really would not work, the individual readily admitted that he was using a new procedure and a new instrument, both of which were probably only 10 percent developed, but insisted that since randomization was what NIH would fund, he was determined to use randomization. Dr. Fogarty declined to participate, but he soon heard from numerous colleagues at other institutions who had not declined, simply because they were going to get paid for it. Here, he concluded, was an early, early stage evolving technology that everybody wanted to document and develop, but they were doing it by the wrong clinical trial method. His question then, for Dr. Watson and NIH, was whether it was not possible to take a parallel path to address the issue.

Dr. Watson agreed that researchers need to think more about those things up front, in some collective way, and get back to what he called guidance sections that work on trial design for this class of devices and give guidance up front. Although he said he is a very strong advocate of randomization from the very first patient, for a variety of reasons, there is an example similar to Fogarty's with ventricular assist systems, where there have now been several studies conducted. A major meeting has been organized by the American College of Cardiology to look at what has happened and see whether researchers ought to employ different clinical designs.

Susan Alpert from the FDA volunteered that something else very important is involved, and that is that the clinical community is at the table for a lot of these discussions pushing the idea that the technology actually is ready. They are using the technology in ways that may or may not be appropriate and are actually forcing the initiation of the trials. That is, the clinical community is pulling the technology forward rather than waiting for it or working with an individual company. Dr. Alpert opined that it is the duty of everyone in the medical device community and the clinical community, not just the government, to protect patients. One of the suggestions that has been brought up today, she said, is to do uncontrolled trials to start, to do registry trials as the only trials, but that presents many difficulties. Researchers then never can ethically do the trial that actually answers the question as to how one technology compares to another because by the time the device has been used with 2,000 or 3,000 people under a registry, the same investigators state that it is unethical to do a randomized trial because they already have the answer. We have to clarify how technologies are to be developed, who is at the table as they are being developed, and how to more quickly obtain the small amounts of information that are needed in a focused setting rather than with thousands of people in a registry. Do a focused first cut if that is needed and then get those randomized trials started because they are the ones that are crucial. They are going to answer the question, not just for marketing, but for reimbursement as well.

Kshitij Mohan from Baxter International suggested that the issue with respect to clinical trials is a broader one of what is appropriate science for the validation of technology. For example, if the concern is durability, should that be evaluated on an engineering bench or in clinical trials? Obviously one is more appropriate, depending on the question. If a chip has been already validated to failure rates of 1 in 10^{12}, little additional information about that chip will be gained through a clinical trial. With that in mind, Dr. Mohan suggested that some outcomes research on the regulatory process itself should be done. He cited the tremendous amount of data available in the 5,000 or so premarket notifications (510(k)s) submitted to FDA each year over the last two decades, the 40 or 50 premarket approval applications (PMAs) submitted each year, and the tens of thousands of medical device reports (MDRs) on failures and malfunctions. Shouldn't there be some work done, he asked, some systematic research into what validation tools yield the greatest value in terms of demonstration of safety, effectiveness, or economic value with respect to reimbursement?

Dr. Alpert pointed out that the PMA process and the clinical trials process are for unproven technologies, for real innovation where no answers are available, while 510(k)s are for incremental changes to proven technology. It is nevertheless very important to think about which aspects should be measured. Which aspects belong in a clinical trial to establish safety and effectiveness and impact on patients and which aspects of a technology actually are better tested at the bench?

Thomas Loarie, CEO of Kera Vision, offered the view from a smaller company with limited resources. Their cornea-shaping technology is apparently being considered by some surgeons in Europe for use in treating keratoconus, a bulging of the cornea that is estimated to afflict 1 out of 2,000 people and often necessitates a corneal transplant. When a doctor in Europe approached him a few years ago, Loarie told him not to do it, for fear that it might affect their PMA in the queue at FDA. Anything that happens with the product must be reported to the FDA, so some doctor going off and doing something that the product was never designed for could jeopardize the company's entire investment. Doctors do not usually listen to people who run companies, Loarie continued, and six months to a year later he saw the same doctor in Paris, who reported that he had been treating six patients for keratoconus and had completely stopped the disease progression. He and some colleagues have now organized a physician-type investigational device exemption (IDE) trial to get more data, and Kera Vision has started getting more pressure to run formal trials both in Europe and in the United States. The problem is that they cannot afford it. It may be a great breakthrough for keratoconus, but the company just cannot afford to run a trial on a such a rare disease as keratoconus.

Dr. Alpert pointed out that there is nothing wrong with European data. If the studies are studies conducted appropriately, the data are perfectly acceptable to the FDA. However, she agreed that the cost of clinical trials in this country is an extremely important topic, especially the cost of overhead from the major academic institutions. There are some new tools, alternatives to clinical trials to support these things, she asserted, not perfect tools, but there are more tools. Researchers need to allow development of technology, she continued, but under the right controls that protect patients, and if they do not have all the tools, then they ought to be developing them.

Jim Benson pointed out that there are indeed such tools, humanitarian exemptions, treatment with investigational new drugs (INDs), IDEs, and postmarket coverage as opposed to premarket data, but what is often missing is knowledge on the part of a company that has an issue like this that they can, in fact, have those discussions

Robert Califf of Duke University promised to address academic overhead and costs of clinical trials in his afternoon talk, because, as he put it, there is no shortage of innovative ideas. It is the funding to actually get the necessary data that is in short supply. As a clinical trialist responding to Dr. Fogarty, Dr. Califf claimed that a lot of devices have gone down the tubes because of well-intentioned inventors who did not know the basic fundamentals of clinical research. He pointed to gene therapy, where once again very intelligent people just did not know the fundamentals of what one must do when doing a human experiment.

Dr. Califf also raised an ethical question regarding overseas clinical trials. What one calls clinical trials or device development, he said, is a human experiment. The idea of saying it is too hard to do in the United States, so researchers will do the experiments on human beings in Europe, raises a lot of issues that really need thought by many people. Europeans are no more expendable in terms of experimentation than Americans.

Califf went on to say that anyone who has worked with devices or done research with devices knows that the fundamental questions are who should be allowed to tinker, and how far can one go with tinkering before it is a new experiment that demands informed consent and reporting of what one is doing.

Researchers have evolved from the 1970s, when any doctor who wanted to fiddle with something could pretty much do it, to a year 2000 in which if a doctor changes the size of a urological catheter in a standard procedure for more than three or four people and writes a case series in a journal, he risks censure for doing human subjects research without the approval of an Institutional Review Board.

Mr. Loarie responded by noting that his company had started its investigational work in Brazil and done further research in Mexico and in Europe, and he had yet to meet a doctor in any of those countries who was unconcerned about harm to a patient. Integrity of clinical research is not unique to the United States. These doctors have practices. They have reputations and they demand a lot from Loarie's company before they will do anything.

Dr. Alpert brought the discussion to a close by noting that FDA actually addressed the issue of tinkering during clinical trials. Devices are allowed to evolve during clinical trials, despite the implication yesterday that nothing can be changed. During an IDE, a product can, in fact, evolve appropriately as long as impact of the changes on the data is taken into consideration, that is, the ability to pool data to understand what that technology or that technological change or the tinkering or the modification of manufacturing has accomplished.

Obviously, communication is very important, but there is opportunity for products to evolve during clinical trials and not be absolutely frozen. There are formulation issues in dealing with drugs, and there are changes in device design that can, in fact, render the data non-poolable. That must be considered as one goes forward but one can, in fact, evolve.

5

The Challenges Ahead

In this session, speakers examined the challenges that lie ahead for medical device innovation, such as identifying areas of clinical medicine in which there are significant unmet needs. Speakers discussed emerging discoveries and technologies that could serve as the basis for developing new medical devices, addressing clinical needs, improving costs, or bettering outcomes of currently available devices.

UNMET CLINICAL NEEDS: CARDIOVASCULAR DISEASE
James E. Muller, M.D.
Center for Integration of Medicine and Innovative Technology

Cardiovascular disease is the largest single cause of medical morbidity and mortality in the United States. It is responsible for over 1.5 million myocardial infarctions annually and over 200,000 sudden cardiac deaths. In addition, the problem of congestive heart failure is one of the leading causes of expenditures for hospitalization.

With progress that has been made in the basic sciences and engineering, it is quite feasible to envision improved devices that are not only more effective but also improve the cost-effectiveness of cardiovascular care. There are many opportunities to extend the use of devices and to improve devices for cardiovascular purposes.

As currently practiced, cardiovascular surgery generally involves thoracotomy, which causes significant morbidity for patients and prolonged hospital stays. There is an unmet need for methods to perform coronary artery bypass grafting without the need for a full thoracotomy. There are numerous "minimally invasive" approaches that have been taken to bypass surgery and the area is one of rapid experimentation and development.

One method that may be useful is that of robotic-assisted, coronary artery bypass grafting. With advanced technology and computer systems it is now possible for a surgeon to manipulate sensors and effectors that permit the anastomosis of an internal mammary artery to the left anterior descending coronary artery without the need for a thoracotomy. Research on such a technique is underway at several institutions and robotic-assisted, coronary artery bypass grafting has been performed in living patients in Europe. This is an area in which further device development is expected and needed.

A method has also been proposed to perform coronary artery bypass grafting of total coronary occlusions with the use of the neighboring coronary vein. This method has been developed by Dr. Stephen Oesterle, formerly of Stanford University, and has been entitled percutaneous in situ coronary artery bypass grafting (PICAB). The PICAB method utilizes an approach through the femoral vein, involving puncture of the coronary vein adjacent to the left anterior descending coronary artery. Both distal and proximal punctures are made around a 100% stenosis. Connections are then made to the coronary vein, and the vein is blocked both distal and proximal to the conduit portion. This method could make it possible to perform bypass without the need for thoracotomy.

In addition to the methods mentioned above to treat stenosis, there is an urgent need to identify and treat plaques that are not stenotic but that are vulnerable to rupture. Such plaques are the most frequent cause of myocardial infarction and sudden cardiac death. There are multiple technologies capable of characterizing tissue that could be utilized for these purposes. Optical coherence tomography (OCT) has been successfully utilized to obtain very high-resolution images of coronary tissue in living patients. It is also possible to utilize near infrared spectroscopy, both diffuse reflectance and Raman forms, to identify the chemical composition of tissue. Other techniques proposed to identify vulnerable plaque include increased temperature detection, and, in non-invasive tests, ultra fast CT, and magnetic resonance imaging. From this broad range of technology and potential devices, it is highly likely that plaques vulnerable to rupture can be identified before they rupture. This could permit randomized trials of numerous types of plaques stabilization therapy that could be developed.

An additional area in which device development is needed is that of electrophysiology. New forms of energy delivery including radio frequency, thermal, and photonic-based energy sources are under development for the ablation of tracts that cause arrhythmia.

In summary, the cardiovascular area is one of major importance because of the severity and prevalence of cardiovascular disease. The diseases that are causing the major morbidity and mortality for the country in the cardiovascular area are amenable to therapy with a broad range of devices that can definitely be improved, given the current level of development of technology.

UNMET CLINICAL NEEDS: CLINICAL TRIALS
Robert Califf, M.D.
Associate Vice Chancellor for Clinical Research
Duke University

The most important unmet need right now is clinical information systems that will provide information about whether devices are effective and cost-saving. Researchers need rational information that can help them make informed judgments that are ultimately for the best of all involved.

Gathering evidence is a challenge. For example, treatment effects are almost always modest. In addition, studies have to be done in the sickest patients to get measurable treatment effects, which raises procedural and ethical issues. Unintended effects are very common, especially when products are combined in a single patient. This is a special problem for devices because the other interaction is between the device itself and the human being who is using the device. This has major implications for the way clinical trials are conducted, especially since it can be difficult to sort out adverse events that are due to the device rather than the underlying condition or interactions with other drugs or devices.

While it is easy to be critical of the inventor/investigator and the tinkering that goes on, it is also fair to say that right now researchers are pretty much in their infancy in terms of really understanding how to construct accurate assessment of risk and benefit, even when the raw data are high quality. Without good data, it is almost impossible to construct reasonable evidence-based perspectives on how patients should be treated. Unless researchers develop better methods of keeping practitioners educated and informed and building systems to help them practice, the best inventions in the world are not going to have much of an impact on the public health. This is evidenced in part by the continued—almost unbelievable—variation in the way that medical devices are used. Researchers have no hope of really detecting the kind of important differences that are needed unless they really study them with adequate methodology, and with adequate sample sizes.

Five issues face clinical trials of medical devices: informed consent versus tinkering, incentive versus protection from conflict of interest, global markets and standards versus global regulatory standstills, access to medical products versus avoidance of risk, and evolutionary innovation versus regulation.

If researchers had ways of collecting the data so they did not spend all the venture capital raised trying to do the clinical trials, one could spend more of it on working on the inventions. The medical profession is going to be forced *to develop common clinical data systems* that use common nomenclatures so that researchers can ensure the public that they are maintaining privacy and that they know what they are talking about when they prescribe therapies over the long term.

Imagine a system where there really were Web-based point-of-care clinical information systems, where doctors use the same names for the same things, with personal patient records that were transportable, where the data could be harvested and aggregated in think tanks. If one had a new device and wanted to try it out or test it one would not have to spend a fortune building a clinical data system and paying clinical research organizations and academic centers to deal with all these regulations and collect all these data.

BARRIERS AND ISSUES IN DEVICE INNOVATION: REIMBURSEMENT
Pamela Bailey
President, Health Industry Manufacturers Association[1]

The role of the Health Industry Manufacturers Association (HIMA) is to be an advocate for innovation and to help its member companies move through the regulatory and public policy processes. Because regulation is the result of legislation to affect change either in the regulatory process or within public policy, researchers all need to be players in the broader policy and political debates. For example, FDA is given a budget by Congress, and researchers want to make sure it is adequate for FDA to fulfill its mission.

Other issues of prime importance are access to global markets and adequate coverage, globally and in the United States, and adequate payment. Reimbursement and coverage, whether it is at the managed care site or whether it is by Medicare, is like a dark, winding, country road through the woods with no road signs. Over 140,000 pages of regulations embody Medicare. The combination of regulation and payment barriers creates uncertainty, which is a barrier to innovation.

In terms of its process for handling the medical devices industry in processing and accelerating technology, Medicare does not innovate. This means that many technologies take years after they are cleared by FDA to be available to the patient and the impact on the patient and on patient care is clear. Delays in assignments of payment codes to FDA-approved products is a tremendous barrier raised by HCFA.[2] Even when codes are assigned after long delays, the amount of reimbursement considered acceptable by HCFA can be disastrously low for the innovator. HCFA has begun some reform of the coverage process, but there is only so much they can do. Legislation has to be passed to really fix the process.

A crucial problem is that no one has a clear sense of data requirements for proving whether a device is cost-effective or how to adequately demonstrate outcomes or clinical effectiveness for the purposes of payment.

Recent legislation considerably reforms the inherent reasonableness authority and the way new technologies, and particularly more expensive innovative technologies, are reimbursed in the outpatient setting. This is a significant achievement because it was a collaborative effort among industry, Congress, and HCFA. Researchers are hopeful that they can use some of that methodology to begin to work on the inpatient setting, particularly in terms of making it easier

---

[1] Now Advanced Medical Technology Association (AdvaMed).
[2] Now Centers for Medicare and Medicaid Services (CMS).

for newer technology to be covered and to be adequately paid for so that there are incentives to develop new technology.

GENERAL DISCUSSION OF THE CHALLENGES AHEAD

David Feigal of FDA opened the discussion by commenting on the synchronization of FDA and HCFA mentioned by Pamela Bailey. He described some recent discussions between FDA and HCFA about imaging innovation for cancer detection and evaluation of extent of cancer, which he characterized as one of the few public forums where FDA and HCFA and companies and NIH have actually all been at the table at the same time. One of the topics that comes up at such meetings is why FDA approval is not good enough for reimbursement. There is apparently a perception that, even in the approval of drugs where clinical trials are much more uniformly required, the evidence that FDA gets does not always address a clinical benefit. HCFA's mandate, said Feigal, is to look for the value added for their recipients. They are shepherding their recipients' dollars, which come from their taxes and our taxes. For example, they sometimes will be evaluating a new product comparatively, whereas FDA regulations never require that one establishes one's comparative efficacy. In fact, FDA usually prefers placebo controls, where that is still ethical.

More to the point for the device industry, said Feigal, are products that come in under 510(k) (premarket notifications of intent to market a product that is substantially equivalent to one already legally marketed) without any clinical data, are judged substantially equivalent, and are approved based on performance standards. FDA does not think that those products do not have clinical benefit; they are just linking them to things that have already demonstrated a benefit. But if HCFA then asks the manufacturer of the new medical device to show clinical trial data, all the manufacturer can say is that these performance standards were met and this is how the product is linked to other products. Similarly, even within the same product class over time, FDA is allowed to decrease requirements and down-classify products, but then HCFA may look at them and demand data on clinical benefits.

A second point raised by Dr. Feigal concerned the notion that the path to the market is a linear one with everything done in a specific order. Difficult as it is to contemplate deciding on reimbursement at the same time as deciding a code, Feigal claimed that FDA is willing to start the discussions about how to do that. One of the quirks of fate is that the Center for Devices has been given the responsibility to be the liaison to HCFA for all of FDA, and they are eager to work on these problems with HCFA and industry.

Pamela Bailey agreed that HCFA could learn much from FDA, but also pointed out that one of the options for reforming Medicare is to establish it almost totally in a private plan choice option, which would put the technology assessment much more in the context of what is done with private managed care or insurance plans today. There would still be a traditional HCFA, but it would be a much smaller component when it comes to assessing technology. She challenged the clinicians in the audience, or even some of the companies, to comment on how they find the route to market when it goes through a private managed care plan rather than through Medicare. She believes that companies will be the first to say that they have not all figured it out yet either, but in many ways the care plans are much easier to deal with because they are smaller and they have a different set of incentives than HCFA. Nevertheless, she concluded, more and more industry is coming to recognize that when they talk about innovation, it is not just FDA, but the payment folks have to be brought in as well.

Robert Califf of Duke University brought up the perception of care providers that anything can be listed and added at a price, but when they add up the cost of providing care relative to what researchers get paid, and Medicare is actually pretty generous compared to most managed care now, available or not, they just cannot afford to do it. Ms. Bailey echoed Dr. Califf's concern, noting that that is just why HCFA has to deal with the cost of technology.

Percy Bridger from HCFA pointed out that the 1989 proposed regulations for coverage criteria are just not going to be applicable to today's world, and a lot of that has to do with the discussions surrounding costs. In fact, he said, HCFA works under a system that was developed and enacted in 1965, a system that does not really work so well in the year 2000.

Jeff Lerner from ECRI explained that he often does HCFA technology assessments for the private sector, and gets into a dilemma. Industry often asks him why he does not tell them what the standards are for evaluation, but they also tell him to be careful not to retard innovation. Lerner's response has generally been that it is not easy to do both. One cannot necessarily say how a device will be evaluated, because if each technology is to be treated on its own merits, it must be evaluated in a unique way. If all technologies are treated exactly the same way, innovation winds up getting cut off. It is impossible to have it both ways. In a routinized process somebody always loses. If the evaluation process is individualized, then it is impossible to specify the evaluation standards in advance.

Dr. Califf complimented the FDA for having standards, but always saying that if one sees that a product is going to be different, come in and talk about it and a different plan will be accepted. He pointed out, however, that all the agencies around the world do not always agree on criteria for negotiation. It seems to work pretty well for companies that go in ahead of time and make the case. So, in a way researchers do have it both ways, but that requires thought about the nature of the assessment. Nevertheless, he concluded, maybe some of the things FDA has done, if adopted by HCFA, would speed things up quite a bit and still be fair.

Dr. Lerner brought up the idea of journals exclusively for industry-supported research, where it is clear that the work is from industry and everyone can agree on certain checks on the research. Right now there is a system of journals in which, he said, one is supposed to hide the fact that research might be supported by industry.

Dr. Califf responded that research should not be characterized as either industry or academic, although affiliations do need to be acknowledged, and biases and conflicts made public. He conceded that there probably is a way to go with this idea, particularly with some topics. Cost-effectiveness analysis is the most controversial, but in his own field of cardiovascular disease, he estimated that the vast majority of good research is industry-funded, and oftentimes that work is more creative, easier, and more effective because of the absence of all those committees that want to change everything the investigator is trying to accomplish.

Mr. Lerner amplified on his earlier thought by pointing out that one can have both, but there should not be a system where one has to pretend that is not going on because that leads to subterfuges. As evidence he cited the Krimsky studies out of Tufts, which, he said, looked at 62,000 articles for conflict-of-interest disclosures and found that only 0.5 percent of them contained any statement of author personal financial interests.

Dr. Califf agreed that there is a problem. His analysis was that two trends are contributing. One is industry authors who do not acknowledge that fact out of concern that it would lead to a lower evaluation. The other is the professional writing company, where the authors listed actually do not even know what is in the paper.

Robert Anderson of Duke suggested that the manufacturers and HIMA have to take a look at these practices as well as academia, and that perhaps they ought to have an institutional review board. He recalled his experience on a surgery and biomedical engineering study section, where they would get hundreds of grants, 50 percent of which could be thrown out almost immediately as absolute garbage. He suggested that one of the reasons the FDA and HCFA may be so swamped is that they try and treat everything equally; they do not have the right to triage and cull out the obviously poor proposals. Perhaps, he continued, HIMA or some independent group could have an IRB to look at proposals destined for FDA and decide whether they are worth someone at FDA spending time on.

Peter Bouxsein of HCFA declined to speak for HCFA, but reminded the group that HCFA and FDA are asked very different questions. FDA is asked whether it is reasonable to put this product into commerce. Will the public be protected at a certain level of safety, and will the product do what it is designed to do so that people can make a decision whether to use it? FDA carries out that mission in a very appropriate way.

HCFA is asked a completely different question. The product has already been approved by FDA as safe and effective enough for public commerce. HCFA takes the role of purchaser and copes with the question of whether it is sensible to buy this product. HCFA is representing beneficiaries, including the economic interest of beneficiaries, and the economic interest of the American public and the taxpayers.

Bouxsein closed the session with an anecdote about Uwe Reinhardt that illustrates this difference in the roles of FDA and HCFA. Reinhardt once told an audience like this one that they may not realize it but there are two ways of doing a tonsillectomy, both equally effective. They achieve the same result, the same outcomes, the same risk, but one is far more elegant than the other and costs 20 times as much. Reinhardt asked, "What should HCFA do? Should they just go ahead and pay for both of them or should they make a decision to pay for the cheaper one and not for the more expensive one?" Then he stopped. The audience, of course, was on the edge of their seats saying, well, what is the second procedure. Finally they could not take anymore and called out for Uwe to please tell them what is the second procedure. "Oh", he said, "I thought you knew. It is transurethral."

6

Summary and Conclusions

Kshitij Mohan, Ph.D.
Workshop Chair

Science and technology developments are no longer sequential events. A myriad of changes are occurring in the device development and approval process, including the use of computers, e-mail, teleconferencing and the internet; high- throughput screening, rational drug design, bioengineering and miniaturization; more concern about special populations, including children, the elderly, and women; and greater access to products at their investigational stage. The medical device life cycle is not a simple, linear progression from basic to applied research, to development, to marketing. Rather, it is a complex stream of five parallel tracks involving regulation, research and development, marketing, manufacturing, and legal issues.

There are new challenges in the processes of technology integration and transfer, notably long lead times and the need for many iterations. This tests the adaptability of academia and industry to come up with new models of parallel discovery, development, and economics. FDA has responded by speeding up its regulatory approvals but there will always be new tests of the science behind the regulation. Researchers can no longer adhere to the dogma that there is only one way to test new clinical devices. There is room for continual improvement in the science and in the guidance given to those trying to get new devices through the regulatory process to market. In such guidance, researchers need to determine the appropriate level of transparency and clarity necessary to permit wide application across many types of devices.

Public and private financial resources are available in the field of devices, but such sources are limited and often unpredictable. The Small Business Innovation and Research Program created in the early 1980s is an underused federal source of funds for device company startups. Underuse of this opportunity is especially unfortunate at a time when 52% of the teaching hospitals in this country are running at a loss. These medical centers are often the source of innovation in the medical device arena. Industry funds much of the innovative work going on in academe. This is a positive influence, and journals and academicians should be forthcoming about the role of private funds in the research and development process.

Researchers also need better mechanisms for quickly establishing reimbursement policies for investigative devices. The basic issue here is: what is the methodology for evaluating the costs, benefits, and values of new devices? This should not be a difficult task given the relatively small contribution of devices to the overall health services environment. The Health Care Financing Administration (HCFA),[1] the Veterans Administration, and FDA should get together and address these issues.

Public forums in which FDA, HCFA, the National Institutes of Health (NIH), and companies sit at the same table would be one way of improving the reimbursement dilemma. Such a forum would allow agencies such as HCFA to have a greater sense of the value added by a technology. Approval by FDA of a device's safety and efficacy is only one step toward the marketplace. HCFA's responsibility is to represent the beneficiaries, including their economic interests, as well as the economic interest of the American public and the taxpayers. The device industry must be more proactive in approaching HCFA early on in the process.

There are a number of ways in which the regulatory process for devices is improving, including the use of advisory groups, either in public forums or in private sessions; streamlining the process, particularly with respect to second- and third-generation devices; expedited reviews for breakthrough, highly beneficial innovations; early interactions and consultations on new, high-impact products; reducing burdens on companies with an excellent track record; increased access, particularly for smaller companies; facilitating access to and coordination with NIH and HCFA; and better coordination within FDA with respect to combination products.

---

[1] Now Centers for Medicare and Medicaid Services.

Appendix A

Workshop Agenda
Roundtable on Research and Development of Drugs, Biologics, and Medical Devices

INNOVATION AND INVENTION IN MEDICAL DEVICES
17–18 FEBRUARY 2000
WYNDHAM CITY CENTER HOTEL
1143 NEW HAMPSHIRE AVENUE, N.W.
WASHINGTON, D.C.

AGENDA

Thursday, 17 February

7:30 a.m. **Continental Breakfast**

Opening Session

8:00   **Welcome and Opening Remarks**
          Kenneth I. Shine, M.D., President
          Institute of Medicine

8:15   **Statement of Objectives, Charge to Participants, Introductions**
          Ronald W. Estabrook, Ph.D., Roundtable Chair
          Virginia Lazenby O'Hara Professor of Biochemistry
          University of Texas Southwestern Medical Center

8:30   **Opening Remarks**
          Kshitij Mohan, Ph.D., Workshop Chair
          Corporate Vice President for Research and Technical Services
          Baxter Health Care Corporation

8:45 **Plenary Speaker**
Harry M. Jansen Kraemer, Jr.
Chairman and Chief Executive Officer
Baxter International, Inc.

Keynote Session

Innovation and invention-related perspectives of key stakeholders (research, clinical practice, regulatory, industry, and consumer constituencies) in the area of medical devices. Past, present, and future directions in medical devices.

Moderator: Ronald W. Estabrook, Ph.D., Roundtable Chair

9:30 **Robert W. Mann, Sc.D.**
Whitaker Professor Emeritus of Biomedical Engineering
Massachusetts Institute of Technology

9:50 **David W. Feigal, M.D., M.P.H.**
Director, Center for Devices and Radiological Health
Food and Drug Administration

10:30 **Tobias Massa, Ph.D.**
Executive Director, Global Regulatory Affairs
Lilly Research Laboratories

10:50 **Jeffrey C. Lerner Ph.D.**
Vice President for Strategic Planning
ECRI

11:10 **Glen D. Nelson, M.D.**
Vice Chairman
Medtronic, Inc.

11:30 **Panel Discussion Period**

Session I: The Nature of Medical Innovation

Presentations in this session will provide the status of innovation in medical devices since the late 1980s, address the invention and development process map for medical device technologies and products, present case studies that analyze the factors which have led to significant medical device innovations in the past 50 years, and discuss the factors that have supported significant ongoing and emerging technology innovations to reach the development and clinical stage.

Moderator: Annetine C. Gelijns, Ph.D.
Director, International Center for Health Outcomes and Innovation Research
Columbia University

APPENDIX A 73

1:30 p.m. **Introductory Comments**
Annetine C. Gelijns, Ph.D.

1:50 **The Innovation Process for Medical Devices: A NASA Perspective**
John Hines, M.S.
Technology Development Manager
Space Life Sciences Program, NASA

2:10 **Case Studies of Significant Medical Device Innovation in the Past**
Thomas J. Fogarty, M.D.
Professor of Surgery
Stanford University School of Medicine

2:30 **Case Studies of Significant Emerging Innovations**
Stephen P. A. Fodor, Ph.D.
Chairman and Chief Executive Officer
Affymetrix

3:10 **Inhaled Insulin—A Case Study**
Robert B. Chess
Chief Executive Officer
Inhale Therapeutics

3:30 **Case Studies of Significant Emerging Innovations**
Richard Nadeau, Ph.D.
Chairman and Chief Executive Officer
Cytometrics

3:50 **Case Studies of Significant Emerging Innovations**
Dean Kamen
President
DEKA Research and Development Corporation

4:10 **Panel Discussion Period**

5:10 **Adjournment**

Friday, 18 February

8:15 a.m. **Opening Remarks**
Ronald Estabrook, Ph.D., Roundtable Chair

Session II: Sources and Support of Medical Device Innovation

Presentations in this session will analyze the sources and amount of resources available in the medical device innovation field; discuss the role of small, large, and multinational medical companies and identify the issues and opportunities confronted by them in this field, as well as the role of standards and product applications; identify the role as well as the incentives and drivers of venture capital; and discuss the role of the legal system.

Moderator: **James S. Benson**
Executive Vice President, Technology and Regulatory Affairs
Health Industry Manufacturers Association

8:30 **An Overview of Public and Private Factors Affecting Medical Device Innovation**
Cliff Goodman, Ph.D.
Senior Scientist
The Lewin Group

8:55 **The Federal Research Role**
John T. Watson, Ph.D.
Acting Deputy Director,
National Heart, Lung and Blood Institute, NIH

9:15 **The Federal Regulatory Role**
Susan Alpert, M.D., Ph.D.
Director, Center for Food Safety and Applied Nutrition
Food and Drug Administration

9:35 **The Academic Role in Innovation**
John A. Parrish, M.D.
Center for Innovative Minimally Invasive Technology
Massachusetts General Hospital

10:20 **The Academic Role**
Robert W. Anderson, M.D.
David C. Sabiston Professor and Chair
Department of Surgery
Duke University

10:40 **Role of Small Medical Companies**
Thomas M. Loarie
Chief Executive Officer
Kera Vision, Inc.

11:00 **Role of Large Medical Companies**
John P. Wareham
Chief Executive Officer
Beckman Coulter

11:20 **Role of Public and Private Capital**
J. Casey McGlynn
Partner—Wilson, Sonsini, Goodrich and Rosati

APPENDIX A 75

11:40 **Panel Discussion Period**

| **Session III: The Challenges Ahead** |

Session III will examine the challenges that lie ahead for medical device innovation, such as identifying areas of clinical medicine where there are significant unmet clinical needs that may be addressed through innovation in medical technology and through training and education, as well as identifying new initiatives in interdisciplinary science for promoting new models for the conduct of research essential to the undergirding of future medical technology. This session will also discuss emerging discoveries and technologies that could serve as the basis for developing new medical devices, addressing the unmet clinical needs, or for improving costs or outcome of currently available devices, as well as identify the potential barriers for present and future technologies which are being applied to medical devices and identify the public perception of risk assessment.

Moderator: Robert Califf, M.D., Roundtable Member
Associate Vice Chancellor for Clinical Research
Duke University

1:30 p.m. **Unmet Clinical Needs**
Robert Califf, M.D.

1:55 **Unmet Clinical Needs**
James E. Muller, M.D.
Center for Innovative Minimally Invasive Therapy

2:20 **Barriers and Issues in Device Innovation: Reimbursement**
Pamela G. Bailey
President, Health Industry Manufacturers Association

2:45 **Panel Discussion Period**

| **Summary and Conclusions** |

3:30 **Summary and Conclusions**
Kshitij Mohan, Ph.D., Workshop Chair

4:00 **Closing Remarks**
Ronald Estabrook, Ph.D., Roundtable Chair

4:20 **Adjournment**

Appendix B

Speakers' Biographical Sketches

Susan Alpert, M.D., Ph.D., is Vice President, Regulatory Sciences at C.R. Bard, a mid-sized medical device company in Murray Hill, New Jersey, where she is responsible for the oversight of quality assurance and regulatory and medical affairs. Prior to this she was the Director of the Food Safety Initiative at the FDA's Center for Food Safety and Applied Nutrition. She previously served as Director of the Office of Device Evaluation (ODE) at the Center for Devices and Radiological Health, FDA, which is responsible for the pre-market evaluation of the safety and effectiveness of medical devices. Dr. Alpert joined the FDA in 1987 as a Medical Officer in the Division of Anti-Infective Drug Products in the Center for Drug Evaluation and Research, where she also served as a supervisor for anti-infective and dermatological drug products. Dr. Alpert received her A.B. in biology from Barnard College, Columbia University, and her Ph.D. in medical microbiology from New York University School of Medicine. She earned her M.D. at the University of Miami School of Medicine, trained in Pediatrics at Montefiore Hospital, Albert Einstein College of Medicine in New York, and completed her training in Pediatric Infectious Diseases at Children's Hospital in Washington, D.C. as part of a joint program with the FDA.

Robert W. Anderson, M.D., is the Chief of Staff of the Duke University Medical Center. In addition, he is Professor and Chairman of Surgery and Professor of Biomedical Engineering at Duke. Dr. Anderson earned a bachelor's degree in engineering from Duke University and an M.D. from Northwestern University. After serving in the U.S. Army and holding several positions at the Duke University Medical Center, he served as Professor of Surgery at the University of

Minnesota Medical School for five years. He then served as Professor of Surgery and Professor of Biomedical Engineering at Northwestern University Medical School for 10 years, before returning to Duke in 1994. Dr. Anderson is a member of several professional societies and the recipient of several NIH honors and awards.

Pamela G. Bailey is President of the Advanced Medical Technology Association (AdvaMed), a Washington, D.C.-based national trade association and the largest medical technology association in the world. AdvaMed represents more than 800 innovators and manufacturers of medical devices, diagnostic products, and medical information systems. As president, Bailey is responsible for developing and implementing legislative and grassroots policy and communication strategies in the health policy arena in order to ensure patients receive timely access to life-saving, life-enhancing medical technologies throughout the world. Bailey has been involved in health care public policy, government relations, and communications for over 30 years. She has worked in the public and private sectors in support of market-based health care reforms. Prior to joining AdvaMed, Bailey served from 1988 to 1999 as president of the Healthcare Leadership Council (HLC), a group of over 50 health care industry chief executives—leaders from the hospital, health plan, pharmaceutical, technology, and physician/nurse sectors. Initiated in 1988, HLC is the exclusive forum for the leadership of the health care industry to jointly develop policies, plans, and programs to accomplish their goals on public policy issues. During the early 1970s, Bailey was a member of the White House staff, rising from a research assistant to the President to Assistant Director of the Domestic Council. From 1975 to 1981, she was director of government relations for the American Hospital Supply Corporation, and from 1981 to 1983, she was Assistant Secretary for Public Affairs for the Department of Health and Human Services (HHS). She joined the White House staff again in 1983 as Special Assistant to the President and Deputy Director of the White House Office of Public Affairs. In 1987, she was named President of the National Committee for Quality Health Care (NCQHC).

James S. Benson is the Executive Vice President, Technology and Regulatory Affairs, at the Health Industry Manufacturers Association. Prior to joining HIMA in 1993, Mr. Benson held various positions at the Food and Drug Administration, most recently as the Director for the Center for Devices and Radiological Health. In 1988, Mr. Benson was enlisted as Deputy Commissioner, with his appointment as Acting FDA Commissioner following in 1989. He held this position for one year, when he resumed the role of Deputy Commissioner. He received a B.S. degree in civil engineering from the University of Maryland and an M.S. degree in nuclear engineering from the Georgia Institute of Technology. Mr. Benson is a member of the Board of Trustees of the American Society for Artificial and Internal Organs. He also serves on the Institute of Medicine Roundtable on Research and Development of Drugs, Biologics, and Medical Devices, as well as on the National Cancer Institute's Technology Evaluation

Committee. In 1997, Mr. Benson was elected to the Food and Drug Law Institute Board of Advisors. During his time at HIMA, Mr. Benson led the Association's efforts to develop and advocate the Biomaterials Access Assurance Act of 1998 and the FDA Modernization Act of 1997.

Robert M. Califf, M.D., is Associate Vice Chancellor for Clinical Research, Director of the Duke Clinical Research Institute, and Professor of Medicine, Division of Cardiology, at the Duke University Medical Center, Durham, North Carolina. He is also editor of the *American Heart Journal*. Dr. Califf has led a coordinating effort for many of the best-known cardiology trials of recent years, including CAVEAT (Coronary Angioplasty versus Excisional Atherectomy Trial), GUSTO (Global Utilization of Streptokinase and t-PA for Occluded Coronary Arteries, EPIC (Evaluation of c7E3 Fab in Preventing Ischemic Complications of High-Risk Angioplasty, and TAMI (Thrombolysis and Angioplasty in Myocardial Infarction). He graduated from Duke University summa cum laude and Phi Beta Kappa in 1973 and from Duke University Medical School in 1978, where he was selected for Alpha Omega Alpha. He is a certified specialist in internal medicine (1984) and in cardiovascular disease (1986) and a Fellow of the American College of Cardiology (1988). He did his internship and residency at the University of California, San Francisco, and a fellowship in cardiology at Duke University. In conjunction with colleagues at the Duke Databank for Cardiovascular Disease, he has written extensively about clinical and economic outcomes in chronic ischemic heart disease. With Drs. Mark and Wagner he is an editor of *Acute Coronary Care*, 2nd edition. He is a section editor in the *Textbook of Cardiovascular Medicine* and is the author of over 500 peer-reviewed articles.

Robert B. Chess is Chairman of Inhale Therapeutic Systems. Mr. Chess joined Inhale in 1991 as its first non-founder employee, and served as its CEO and then co-CEO until 2000. Mr. Chess was previously the co-founder and President of Penederm, Inc., a dermatological pharmaceutical company focused on improved topical delivery. He has held management positions at Intel Corporation and Metaphor Computer Systems (now part of IBM), and served as a member of President Bush's White House staff. Mr. Chess serves on the Board of Directors and Executive Committee of the Biotechnology Industry Organization, is a member of the Board of Pharsight Corp., and is a trustee of the Committee for Economic Development. Mr. Chess received his B.S. degree in Engineering from the California Institute of Technology and an M.B.A. from Harvard.

Ronald W. Estabrook, Ph.D., received his B.S. degree from Rensselaer Polytechnic Institute and his Ph.D. in biochemistry from the University of Rochester. He has held appointments as Professor of Physical Biochemistry at the University of Pennsylvania and as Virginia Lazenby O'Hara Professor of Biochemistry and Chairman of the Department of Biochemistry at the University of Texas Southwestern Medical School. He has also served as Dean of the Graduate School of Biomedical Sciences at the Dallas campus of the University of Texas.

Dr. Estabrook has co-authored over 260 publications, including the editing of 14 books. He has an honorary Doctor of Medicine from the Karolinska Institut in Stockholm, Sweden, and a Doctor of Science from the University of Rochester.

David W. Feigal, Jr., M.D., M.P.H., is Director, Center for Devices and Radiological Health, Food and Drug Administration. He received his B.S. from the University of Minnesota, his M.D. from Stanford University, and his M.P.H. from the University of California at Davis. He held a joint appointment at the School of Medicine and the School of Dentistry at the University of California, San Francisco, as a member of the Department of Medicine and the Department of Epidemiology and Biostatistics. Dr. Feigal joined the FDA in 1992 and has served in a variety of positions in both CDER and CBER, before assuming his current position. He has served on a number of committees sponsored by the World Health Organization, the National Institutes of Health, the Institute of Medicine, and the Centers for Disease Control and Prevention.

Stephen P.A. Fodor, Ph.D., is currently Chairman and Chief Executive Officer of Affymetrix, Inc. He received his B.S. in Biology and M.S. in Biochemistry from Washington State University, and his Ph.D. in Chemistry from Princeton University. From 1986 to 1989, he was a National Institutes of Health postdoctoral fellow at the University of California, Berkeley, working with Professor Richard Mathies. He joined the Affymax Research Institute in Palo Alto in 1989, where he and colleagues were the first to develop and describe combinatorial chemistry synthesis strategies which they then applied to construct the high- density arrays of peptides and oligonucleotides on small glass substrates (chips). These chips now offer the opportunity for tens of thousands of assays to be carried out and detected in a rapid parallel format. Seminal manuscripts describing this work have been published in *Science* (1991, 1996), *Nature* (1993), and *PNAS* (1993). In 1993, Dr. Fodor co-founded Affymetrix, where the chip technology has been used to synthesize many varieties of high-density oligonucleotide arrays containing tens to hundreds of thousands of DNA probes. In 1992, Dr. Fodor and colleagues received the AAAS Newcomb-Cleveland Award for an outstanding paper published in *Science*. He has received various prizes including the Washington State University Distinguished Alumni Award, the Intellectual Property Owner's Distinguished Inventor of the Year Award, the Chiron Corporation Biotechnology Research Award, the Association for Laboratory Automation Achievement Award, and the Jacob Heskel Gabbay Award in Biotechnology and Medicine. He serves on the Keystone Symposium Board of Directors, as well as on the board of directors of several scientific advisory companies.

Thomas J. Fogarty, M.D., is Professor of Surgery at Stanford University. He received his undergraduate degree in biology from Xavier University in Cincinnati and his M.D. from the University of Cincinnati College of Medicine. Previous positions include President of the Medical Staff, Stanford University, and Director of Cardiovascular Surgery at Sequoia Hospital in Redwood City, California. He has acquired over 70 surgical instrumentation patents, including the

Fogarty balloon embolectomy catheter. He has also founded or co-founded over 20 companies in the medical device or services field and serves as a scientific advisor on the boards of numerous other companies. Dr. Fogarty is a member of the American Board of Surgery and the American Board of Thoracic Surgery, and has published over 200 scientific articles and textbook chapters in the fields of general and cardiovascular surgery. He is past president of the Society for Vascular Surgery (1995) and is president-elect of the International Society for Vascular Specialists. Dr. Fogarty was recently honored to receive The Lemelson Prize for Invention and Innovation (2000) and is a 2001 inductee to the National Inventor's Hall of Fame.

Annetine Gelijns is Director of the International Center for Health Outcomes and Innovation Research, and an Associate Professor of Surgical Sciences in the Department of Surgery, College of Physicians and Surgeons, and the School of Public Health (Health Policy and Management), Columbia University, New York City. Her current research focuses on the factors driving the rate and direction of innovative activity in medicine, academic medical centers, and the diffusion of medical technology, and measuring the clinical and economic outcomes of clinical interventions. She directs the Data Coordinating Center for the NIH-supported REMATCH trial, comparing mechanical assist devices to medical management in end-stage heart failure. Before coming to Columbia in 1993, she directed the Program on Technological Innovation in Medicine at the Institute of Medicine, National Academy of Sciences. From 1983 to 1987, she worked for the Steering Committee on Future Health Scenarios and for the Health Council, The Netherlands. Dr. Gelijns has been a consultant to various national and international organizations, including WHO and OECD. She holds a Ph.D. from the medical faculty, University of Amsterdam, and a bachelor's and master's degree in law from the University of Leyden, The Netherlands.

Clifford Goodman, Ph.D., is a Senior Scientist at The Lewin Group, a health care policy and management consulting firm based in Falls Church, Virginia. Dr. Goodman's methodological expertise involves technology assessment, outcomes research, health economics, decision analytic modeling, and studies pertaining to technological innovation, diffusion, and payment. His experience includes managing projects for an international range of government organizations, pharmaceutical and medical device companies, and professional and industry associations. As a National Research Council Fellow and later as director of the Council on Health Care Technology, he managed a series of technology assessment projects at the Institute of Medicine of the National Academy of Sciences (1982–90). He is a board member of the International Society of Technology Assessment in Health Care and is a Fellow of the American Institute for Medical and Biological Engineering. He did his undergraduate work at Cornell University, received a master's degree from the Georgia Institute of Technology, and earned his doctorate from the Wharton School of the University of Pennsylvania.

John Hines is Technology Development Manager for the NASA Space Life Sciences Fundamental Biology Research Program, which operates within the Office of the Director, Ames Research Center (ARC). He also manages the Advanced Technology Development Project in Biosensor and Biotelemetry development (ATD–B) for the NASA Headquarters Life Sciences Division (HQ Code UL), and coordinates sensor technology issues for the Human Space Life Sciences Program (BioAstronautics), managed at the Johnson Space Center. He also originated and presently serves as Program Executive/Advisor for the Sensors 2000! (S2K!) Program, an Advanced Sensor Systems Technology Development Team operating from within the Life Sciences Division of the Astrobiology and Space Research Directorate at ARC. In 1996, Mr. Hines received the NASA exceptional service medal, highlighting his accomplishments in biosensor, biotelemetry, and space flight hardware development and applications. Prior to his NASA activities, he was a Major in the U.S. Air Force assigned as Deputy Chief of the Information Processing Technology Branch in the Avionics Laboratory at Wright-Patterson AFB, Ohio. From 1977–1986, he managed the ARC Cardiovascular Research Laboratory. Mr. Hines has a B.S. in Electrical Engineering from Tuskegee University and an M.S. in EE/Biomedical Engineering from Stanford University.

Dean Kamen is president and owner of DEKA Research & Development Corporation, a Manchester, New Hampshire-based company specializing in advanced technologies in medical equipment. A physicist, engineer, and inventor, Mr. Kamen holds more than 100 U.S. and foreign patents. His inventions include a wearable infusion pump, a portable home dialysis machine, the cardiovascular Crown stent, a high-performance arthroscopic and laproscopic irrigation pump, and a device that is an integral part of a photopheresis machine for the treatment of cancer. Dean's latest invention, unveiled in 1999, is the Independence 3000 IBOT™ Transporter, which was developed for the disabled community. It allows a seated user to move about at eye-level, climb stairs, and traverse uneven and hilly terrain. Mr. Kamen has received numerous awards in the field of medical devices, including: *Design News Magazine's* Engineer of the Year (1994); Fellow of the American Institute of Medical and Biological Engineering (1994); Kilby Award (1994); Hoover Medal (1995); SPE International John W. Hyatt Service to Mankind Award (1996); and the Heinz Award in Technology, the Economy, and Employment (1998). He was elected to the National Academy of Engineering in 1997.

Harry M. Jansen Kraemer, Jr., is chairman and chief executive officer of Baxter International Inc. Mr. Kraemer joined Baxter in 1982 as director of corporate development. He has held senior positions in both domestic and international operations, including senior vice president and chief financial officer. He was named President of Baxter International in 1997. Before joining Baxter, Mr. Kraemer worked for Bank of America and for Northwest Industries. He currently serves on numerous boards, including Northwestern University, Comdisco, Inc., Science Applications International Corporation, Lawrence University, and the Advisory Board for the J.L. Kellogg Graduate School of Management at Northwestern University. Mr. Kraemer received bachelor's degrees in mathematics and economics from Lawrence University and a master's degree in finance and accounting from the J.L. Kellogg Graduate School of Management.

Jeffrey Charles Lerner, Ph.D., for the past 18 years has served as Vice President for Strategic Planning for ECRI, a nonprofit agency and Collaborating Center of the World Health Organization. ECRI's technology assessment information programs are now used worldwide by ministries of health, U.S. federal agencies (such as the Social Security Administration, the Center for Medicare and Medicaid Services, FDA, and AHRQ), state governments, private health plans (such as Kaiser Permanente), clinical specialty societies (such as the American Academy of Pediatrics), hospitals, and other professional constituencies and by consumers directly. Dr. Lerner is Center Director of an Evidence-based Practice Center funded by the Agency for Healthcare Research and Quality and the Coordinator of the Technical Expert Panel of the National Guideline Clearinghouse (a project sponsored by AHRQ in cooperation with the American Medical Association and the American Association of Health Plans). He is also a member of the Medicare Coverage Advisory Committee (MCAC). Dr. Lerner is former president and current member of the Board of the Health Strategy Network, a society of healthcare planners and managers. He is an associate editor of the *Journal of Ambulatory Care Management* and an Adjunct Senior Fellow of the Leonard Davis Institute of Health Economics of the University of Pennsylvania. Dr. Lerner received his B.A. from Antioch College and his M.A., M.Phil., and Ph.D. from Columbia University. He also studied abroad at St. Andrew's University, Scotland.

Thomas M. Loarie served as chairman and chief executive officer of Kera Vision, Inc., which pioneered a non-laser approach to treat common vision problems that reshapes the cornea by surgically adding materials. Mr. Loarie has 30 years of experience in the medical device industry with direct responsibility for bringing numerous innovative medical technologies to the fields of neurosurgery, interventional neuroradiology, oncology, thoracic and cardiovascular surgery, plastic surgery, general surgery, and ophthalmology. Mr. Loarie previously held senior management positions at American Hospital Supply Corporation (now Baxter Healthcare Inc.) in both the medical specialties and international business sectors, including president of Heyer-Schulte. He also served as an Assistant Professor of Surgery at Creighton University Medical School, lecturing on medical technology and public policy. He was a board member, and Executive Committee member of the Health Industry Manufacturers Association, the founder and chairman of the Medical Device CEO Roundtable, a board member of the California Healthcare Institute, and a member of the Medical Technology Leadership Forum. He also served on the Editorial Advisory Board of the *Medical Device Executive Portfolio*, a professional journal, and on the Medical Industry Advisory Board of *Ophthalmology Times*. Mr. Loarie holds a B.S. degree in engineering from Notre Dame University. In addition, he participated in graduate business studies at the University of Minnesota, University of Chicago, and Columbia University. He has lectured and written extensively on medical technology innovation and its implications for health care public policy, including articles in the *Wall Street Journal, Royal Academy of Engineering World Technology Update*, the *Journal of Applied Manufacturing Systems*, and the *Journal of Refractive Surgery*.

Robert W. Mann, Sc.D., since 1974 Whitaker Professor of Biomedical Engineering and now emeritus, has been engaged in biomedical and rehabilitation engineering research at the Massachusetts Institute of Technology since the late 1950s. His contributions have been recognized by his election to the Institute of Medicine in 1971, the National Academy of Engineering in 1973, and the National Academy of Sciences in 1982. In 1977 he was the recipient of the Gold Medal Award of the American Society of Mechanical Engineers and concurrently was awarded their inaugural H. R. Lissner Award for Outstanding Bioengineering. Other related recognitions include: in 1969 a Citation for Sensory Aids for the Blind from the Associated Blind of Massachusetts, in 1972 an IR-100 Award for the M.I.T. Braillemboss, in 1976 the Goldenson Award for Outstanding Scientific Research in Technology for Cerebral Palsy and the Physically Handicapped, and in 1979 the Engineering Society of New England Award. In 1979–1981 he was Sigma Xi National Lecturer, and in 1980 he was the ALZA Distinguished Lecturer of the Biomedical Engineering Society. He is a fellow of the American Society of Mechanical Engineers, the Institute of Electrical and Electronic Engineers, the American Association for the Advancement of Science, the American Academy of Arts and Sciences, and a founding fellow of the American Institute of Medical and Biological Engineers.

Tobias Massa, Ph.D., is Executive Director, Global Regulatory Affairs, Eli Lilly and Company, responsible for all regulatory aspects of chemistry, manufacturing, and controls for all Eli Lilly products, as well as submission coordination, labeling, and medical information. He is a member of numerous research and corporate executive steering committees in the areas of regulatory affairs, pharmaceutical development and manufacturing, preclinical and clinical research, and labeling. He received his B.A. (cum laude) in chemistry from SUNY at Buffalo and his doctorate in biomedical sciences from the Mt. Sinai School of Medicine (CUNY). He has been a Diplomat of the American Board of Toxicology since 1981. Dr. Massa was a toxicologist at the Schering Plough Research Institute from 1978 to 1986 and was Associate Director/Group Leader in Toxicology for Pfizer from 1986 to 1990. He rejoined Schering Plough as Associate Director of Regulatory Affairs in 1990 and was most recently Senior Director of Worldwide Regulatory Affairs (Chemistry/Manufacturing/Controls) prior to joining Lilly in 1998. Dr. Massa is past chair of the Biology and Biotechnology Committee, and member of the PDUFA III implementation team of the Pharmaceutical Research and Manufacturers of America. He currently chairs PhRMA working groups on site-specific stability, Phase 2/3 CMC IND requirements and manufacturing changes. He is chair of the Product Quality Research Institute Scientific Steering Committee and is a member of the PQRI Board of Directors. He is also past chair of the FDA Committee of the Biotechnology Industry Organization.

J. Casey McGlynn is a partner at Wilson, Sonsini, Goodrich, and Rosati. His practice focuses on the organization, funding, and corporate representation of companies in the information technology and life sciences industries, providing assistance to hundreds of companies in the life sciences, semiconductor, software, and telecommunications sectors. As a strategic business partner, Mr. McGlynn and his group offer focused resources and capabilities to meet the most critical needs of startup and emerging growth companies, including private and venture capital financings, public offerings, university licensing, and strategic collaborations. Mr. McGlynn joined the firm in 1978 and has been a member of the firm's executive, nominating, and compensation committees. He is a frequent contributor to magazines and newsletters focused on angel and venture investing. He is also a frequent speaker on issues relating to the organization and funding of new ventures. Mr. McGlynn received his B.S. and J.D. degrees, with highest honors, from Santa Clara University.

Kshitij Mohan, Ph.D., is Corporate Vice President for Baxter International, Inc. He is responsible for corporate research and technical services, including research centers in the United States and Europe, and for emerging technology ventures and technology strategy development. He is also the founder and leader of the Baxter Technical Council and serves on the Baxter Operating Management Team. Before joining Baxter in 1988, Dr. Mohan was a researcher at the National Bureau of Standards, served in various capacities in the U.S. Food and Drug Administration, and served in the Office of Management and Budget. He also served on two White House task forces and led an inter-agency study of the U.S. Antarctic program. Dr. Mohan has published widely in the fields of health policies, regulations, R&D policies and applied physics, and has lectured and consulted worldwide. He has also served on numerous boards and editorial boards. Dr. Mohan received his Ph.D. in physics from Georgetown University and has extensive training in Management.

James E. Muller, M.D. is a senior member of Center for Integration of Medicine and Innovative Technology, with responsibilities for general CIMIT development and cardiovascular medicine. From 1972 to 1989, Dr. Muller conducted clinical research at the Brigham and Women's Hospital on the triggering of the onset of cardiovascular disease. Prior to joining CIMIT in 1999, he served as Chief of the Cardiovascular Division of the Deaconess Hospital in Boston and subsequently as Director of the Gill Heart Institute in Lexington, Kentucky. He is currently the Director of Clinical Research in the Cardiology Division of the

MGH, Harvard Medical School, and Principal Investigator of a multicenter NIH grant on the triggers of sudden death. Dr. Muller was one of three United States founders of the International Physicians for Prevention of Nuclear War, the organization awarded the 1985 Nobel Peace Prize. He has experience with application of high technology to medicine, through his work as a founder of InfraReDx, a start-up company dedicated to improving health care through photonics.

Richard Nadeau, Ph.D., is the co-founder, chairman, and CEO of Cytometrics, Inc., a medical device company commercializing point-of-care clinical and diagnostic instrument systems that use its patented orthogonal polarization spectral imaging (OPS Imaging) technology, which he co-invented. As recently published in *Nature Medicine*, OPS Imaging provides, for the first time in humans, the ability to easily observe and measure the microcirculatory system and its surrounding tissue. Dr. Nadeau was co-inventor of Dupont's Automatic Clinical Analyzer (aca®) and was responsible for its commercial launch. He has patented seven inventions, including the reference method of determining blood-urea-nitrogen (BUN). Prior to founding Cytometrics, Dr. Nadeau served as president of several medical diagnostics companies. He received his Ph.D. in biochemistry from West Virginia University. He has served in leadership roles for several professional organizations, including as president of the National Committee for Clinical Laboratory Standards, as a member of the Expert Panel on Instrumentation for the International Federation of Clinical Chemistry, and as an advisor to the FDA. Dr. Nadeau also served as a Visiting Research Associate at the University of Pennsylvania's School of Engineering.

Glen D. Nelson, M.D., is Vice Chairman of the Board of Medtronic, Inc. and has been a director since 1980. He joined Medtronic in 1986 as executive vice president and was elected vice chairman in 1988. Prior to joining Medtronic, Dr. Nelson practiced surgery for 17 years and also served as chairman and chief executive officer of American MedCenters, Inc. and chairman, president, and chief executive officer of Park Nicollet Medical Center. He received his A.B. from Harvard College and his M.D. from the University of Minnesota. Dr. Nelson serves on the boards of several organizations, including St. Paul Companies; Carlson Holdings, Inc.; ABS, INC.; the Medical Technology Leadership Forum; and the Johns Hopkins Medicine Board of Visitors.

John A. Parrish, M.D., is the Chairman of the Department of Dermatology at Harvard Medical School (HMS), Chief of the Dermatology Service at Massachusetts General Hospital (MGH), Professor of Dermatology at HMS, and Professor of Health Science and Technology at Massachusetts Institute of Technology (MIT). Although his original training was in internal medicine, dermatology, and clinical research, he has spent the last 20 years conducting and directing basic research in photobiology, biological effects of lasers, and cutaneous biology. Dr. Parrish, in collaboration with Thomas B. Fitzpatrick, M.D., developed a novel treatment of psoriasis (oral psoralen photochemotherapy, or

PUVA) which is now used worldwide. His research group at MGH introduced laser lithotripsy of kidney stones, selective laser therapy of vascular birthmarks and lesions, and novel laser-based diagnosis and treatments of selective cardiovascular disorders and malignancies. Dr. Parrish organized the first, and now the world's largest, multidisciplinary research group to systematically study the basic nature of laser effects on tissues, the Wellman Laboratories of Photomedicine at MGH, of which he is director. Dr. Parrish is also director of the MGH-Harvard Cutaneous Biology Research Center (CBRC), a research center committed to fundamental research in cutaneous biology as broadly defined. Dr. Parrish is also Director of the Partners-MIT-Draper Center for Innovative Minimally Invasive Therapy (CIMIT), a multidisciplinary research and clinical effort to introduce new therapeutic and diagnostic procedures to improve health care. Dr. Parrish has over 300 publications, many of which describe new treatments and diagnostics. He has written eight books, most of which are textbooks, but include a book on baseball, a book on the Vietnam War, and a book for the layperson on skin.

Kenneth I. Shine, M.D., is President of the Institute of Medicine, the National Academies, and Professor of Medicine Emeritus at the University of California, Los Angeles School of Medicine. He is the immediate past Dean and Provost for Medical Sciences at UCLA. He is also currently Clinical Professor of Medicine at the Georgetown University School of Medicine. Dr. Shine received his A.B from Harvard College and his M.D. from Harvard Medical School. A cardiologist and physiologist, Dr. Shine has held appointments as Assistant Professor of Medicine at the Harvard Medical School and Chair of the Department of Medicine at UCLA. He served as Chair of the Council of Deans of the Association of American Medical Colleges in 1991–92 and President of the American Heart Association in 1985–86.

John P. Wareham is chairman, president and chief executive officer of Beckman Coulter, Inc. Wareham became CEO in September 1998 and was named chairman in February 1999. Prior to these changes, he had served as president and chief operating officer) since 1993. During his tenure as president and COO, Wareham successfully managed a corporate restructuring plan that resulted in significantly improved margins for the corporation. He also led an aggressive acquisition strategy that ultimately resulted in the union of Beckman and Coulter as a new industry leader in diagnostics. Wareham joined Beckman Instruments, Inc. in 1984 as Vice President-Diagnostics Systems Group, a position he held through October 1993. In this capacity, he propelled the company's diagnostic business to a leadership position in the clinical laboratory market, making it one of the most profitable entities in the industry. Wareham's move to the company was preceded by a 15-year career with SmithKline. He began there as an operations research analyst and held positions of increasing responsibility, ultimately serving as Director of Business Planning at SmithKline & French Laboratories-Worldwide, and finally, President of Norden Laboratories. Wareham, who holds a bachelor of science degree in pharmacy from Creighton University in Omaha, Nebraska, began his career as a pharmacist in his family's business. He has a master's degree in Business Administration from Washington University in St. Louis. In addition to being a member and chairman of the Beckman Coulter Board of Directors, he is chairman of the Board of Directors of the Advanced Medical Technology Association (AdvaMed), formerly known as the Health Industry Manufacturers Association (HIMA) in Washington, D.C., is a member of the STERIS Corporation Board of Directors, and is also on the Advisory Board for the John Henry Foundation. Additionally, Wareham is a member of the Center for Corporate Innovation in Los Angeles and the University of California, Irvine (UCI) Executive Roundtable.

John T. Watson, Ph.D., is the Director, Clinical and Molecular Division of Heart and Vascular Diseases, National Heart, Lung, and Blood Institute, National Institutes of Health. Dr. Watson came to NIH in 1976 from the University of Texas Health Science Center where he was chairman of the Graduate Study Program in Biomedical Engineering and Assistant Professor of Surgery and Physiology. He has bachelor's (University of Cincinnati) and master's (Southern Methodist University) degrees in mechanical engineering, and earned a doctorate in physiology from the University of Texas at the Southwestern Medical School. Dr. Watson's experience includes 10 years in industry, 10 years in academia, and 25 years in the public sector. His research interests include medical implant design and science, biomaterials, imaging, and heart failure. He is a Founding Fellow of the American Institute of Medical and Biological Engineering and a member of the National Academy of Engineering.

Appendix C
Registered Participants

Lorrie Ballantine
Program Analyst
Health Care Financing
  Administration

Richard I. Barnett
Director, Science and Technology
Hill-Rom

Marilyn Sue Bogner
Chief Scientist
Institute for the Study of Medical
  Error

Eric L. Brennan
Vice President, Clinical Services
Fluidsense Corporation

Richard L. Buck
Commanding Officer
Navy Environment Health Center

Patricia Bull
Division Director in Plans,
  Analysis and Evaluation
U.S. Navy Bureau of Medicine and
  Surgery

Clair Mille Callan
SVP, Office for Professional
  Standards
American Medical Association

Tess Castle
Director, Technology and Regulatory Affairs
Health Industry Manufacturers
  Association

Dennis Chamot
Deputy Executive Director
Commission on Engineering
  and Technical Systems
National Research Council

Blair Childs
Executive Vice President
Planning and Implementation
Health Industry Manufacturers Association.

Michael D. Clayman
Vice President, Global Regulatory Affairs
Eli Lilly and Company

Jeannett Anastasia Colyvas
Researcher
Institute for International Studies
Stanford University

Arthur Combs
Vice President Respiratory Care
Medical Director
Mallinckrodt, Inc.

Jay Crowley
Systems Safety Engineer
Food and Drug Administration

Hal Danby
Senior Vice President
Advanced Technology
Baxter Healthcare

John Durham
Division Director in Plans, Analysis and Evaluation
U.S. Navy Bureau of Medicine and Surgery

Anne Esposito
Health Policy Advisor to Chairman Mike Bilirakis
House Health and Environment Subcommittee

Laura Gallagher-Potter
Scientist, Veterinary Surgeon
Ethicon-Endo-Surgery, Inc.
Surgical Research and Development Department

Ron Geigle
Polidais, LLC

George Giacoia
Special Expert, Center for Research for Mothers and Children
National Institute of Child Health and Human Development

Ann Gosier
Vice President, Government Affairs
Guidant Corporation

Stephen Groft
Director, Office of Rare Diseases
National Institutes of Health

Jean T. Harmon
Senior Advisor for Diabetes
National Institute of Diabetes and Digestive and Kidney Diseases
National Institutes of Health

Kevin A. Harper
Senior Engineer R&D
Ethicon Endo-Surgery

William A. Herman
Director, Division of Physical Sciences
Food and Drug Administration
Center for Devices and Radiological Health

APPENDIX C

Sharon E. Hippler
Health Insurance Specialist
Health Care Financing
  Administration

Richard J. Hodes
Director, National Institute on
  Aging

Jimmy Hsiao
Research Analyst
The Lewin Group

Ed Jenkins
Medical Device Marketing
Ethicon Endo-Surgery, Inc.

Richard Johnson
Director of Sales
Cytometrics, Inc.

Ronald D. Kaye
Human Factors Specialist
FDA Center for Devices and
  Radiological Health

Kenneth F. Kopesky
Vice President
Corporate Compliance and Audit
Medtronic, Inc.

Sue Losch
Associate
Booz-Allen and Hamilton

Charles Liu
Research Assistant
The Lewin Group

Kelly McConville
Medical Service Corps, United
  States Navy
Director of Health Affairs
Office of the Assistant Secretary of
  the Navy
Department of the Navy
ASN (M&RA) Health Affairs

Captain James Moos
Division Director in Plans,
  Analysis and Evaluation
U.S. Navy Bureau of Medicine and
  Surgery

Joel Myklebust
Project Officer
National Institute on Disability and
  Rehabilitation Research

Ronald S. Newbower
Partners Health Care System, Inc.
Vice President for Research Management

Oye Olukotun
Vice President
Medical and Regulatory Affairs
Mallinckrodt, Inc.

Mary Plock
Vice President, Public Affairs
Health Industry Manufacturers
  Association

David Rodbard
Managing Research Scientist
American Institute for Research

Linda Ruckel
Director, Media Relations
Health Industry Manufacturers
  Association

Fatima Sayyid
Research Fellow
Inchoir/Columbia University

Martin E. Schmieg
Executive Vice President
Cytometrics, Inc.

Patricia B. Shrader
Vice President, Corporate
  Regulatory Affairs
Becton Dickinson & Company